ADVENTURES ON THE WATER

ADVENTURES ON THE WATER
THE POWER OF PADDLEBOARDING TO CHANGE LIVES

EDITED BY
JO MOSELEY

Vertebrate Publishing, Sheffield
www.adventurebooks.com

ADVENTURES ON THE WATER

Edited by Jo Moseley

First published in 2025 by Vertebrate Publishing.

VERTEBRATE PUBLISHING, Omega Court, 352 Cemetery Road, Sheffield S11 8FT, United Kingdom. www.adventurebooks.com

Copyright © Jo Moseley and the contributors 2025.

Pages 151–172 constitute a continuation of the copyright information.

Cover illustration © Megan Hall. *www.flotsamprints.com*

Photo on page 178 © Jo Moseley.

Jo Moseley and the contributors have asserted their rights under the Copyright, Designs and Patents Act 1988 to be identified as authors of this work.

A CIP catalogue record for this book is available from the British Library.

ISBN: 978-1-83981-275-0 (Paperback)

ISBN: 978-1-83981-276-7 (Ebook)

ISBN: 978-1-83981-277-4 (Audiobook)

10 9 8 7 6 5 4 3 2 1

All rights reserved. No part of this work covered by the copyright herein may be reproduced or used in any form or by any means – graphic, electronic, or mechanised, including photocopying, recording, taping, or information storage and retrieval systems – without the written permission of the publisher.

Every effort has been made to obtain the necessary permissions with reference to copyright material, both illustrative and quoted. We apologise for any omissions in this respect and will be pleased to make the appropriate acknowledgements in any future edition.

Vertebrate Publishing is committed to printing on paper from sustainable sources.

Printed and bound by CPI Group (UK), Croydon CR0 4YY.

CONTENTS

THE JOY OF SUP Jo Moseley	1
INTRODUCTION Jo Moseley	5
PADDLEBOARDING WITH ORCAS Cal Major	25
SUP SURF IN THE NORTH Heather Peacock	30
PADDLEBOARDING HOME Shilpa Rasaiah	35
CIRCUMNAVIGATING GREAT BRITAIN Brendon Prince	41
SUP YOGA: EMBRACING THE WOBBLE Kathy Marston	46
SUNRISE SUN SALUTATIONS AFTER A STROKE Cathy Miles	51
MOTHER AND SON RACING TOGETHER Anna and James Little	56
FATHER AND DAUGHTER ON THE WATER Dale Mears	62
NORTH OF ORDINARY: YUKON 1000 Scott 'Skip' Innes and Craig Sawyer	66
ANYTHING IS POSSIBLE ON A PADDLEBOARD Caroline Dawson	70
THE EARLY DAYS John Hibbard	75
DESIGNING FOR INCLUSIVE PADDLEBOARDING Will Behenna	79
MAKING A DIFFERENCE Adya Misra	84
HEALING: MY CANCER JOURNEY Melody Smith	87
BLUE HEALTH AND BLUE SPACES Clare Osborn	92

PADDLEBOARDING PODCAST Simon Hutchinson	96
FROM CHAMPION ON THE WATER TO STAR BEHIND THE MIC Sarah Thornely	101
UNEARTHING UNITY Gemma Palmer-Dighton	106
KNOWING WHERE I AM MEANT TO BE Emily King	112
BLUE SPACE HIGHLAND Leeanne MacKay	117
QUEEN OF THE CANALS Daisy Best	122
SUP WITH A PUP Steph Barnicoat	127
SCOTTISH FIVE ISLANDS CHALLENGE Linn van der Zanden	133
EXTREME DREAM TO ST KILDA Dean Dunbar	139
A HEALING JOURNEY Katie Simmons	145
CONTRIBUTORS	151
ABOUT THE EDITOR	177
TOP TIPS	179
ACKNOWLEDGEMENTS	181
FURTHER READING AND LINKS	182

While we have shared the many well-being benefits of stand-up paddleboarding for our physical, mental, social and emotional health, we are not in any way suggesting it is a replacement for proper medical intervention, counselling or medication.

THE JOY OF SUP
JO MOSELEY

Paddleboarding has opened up so many wonderful opportunities and friendships. It has quite literally transformed my life, and I know I am not alone in this experience.

I lie back and look up to the now bright blue sky as the waves gently lap against my paddleboard. Tucked into a sheltered spot along the loch, I close my eyes and feel the warmth of the sun. 'Thank you for this moment,' I say to myself, just as I do every time I go out on to the sea, canal or lake. No one can hear me of course but it is a tiny joyful ritual developed over the last eight years of paddling. I'm creating a memory to tuck away in my heart and soul, ready to draw upon when life feels hard and happiness eludes me.

Today the moment is extra special.

I woke early to write in my journal, appreciating as I did so that without stand-up paddleboarding, I wouldn't be staying on Marie's gorgeous croft on Skye. Lena, the founder of Skye Community Cinema, would not have invited me to join them at the Gathering Hall to speak about beautiful places to SUP and my first two books as part of the Kendal Mountain Tour. I wouldn't have danced my heart out at ceilidh practice nor have said yes to spending Saturday night in Portree at my first roller-skating disco.

Paddleboarding has opened up so many wonderful opportunities and friendships. It has quite literally transformed my life, and I know I am not alone in this experience.

Perhaps if you are reading this book it has happened for you too.

Or maybe your own SUP journey is about to begin. I am thrilled for your adventure ahead.

After a flask of tea as I dangle my legs in the chilly, clear waters, I ready myself to return to my launch spot. It is International Women's Day and Marie and I are going swimming at one of her favourite beaches with friends.

The wind has picked up and is now behind me. I hold my paddle aloft like a sail to catch the breeze and whoosh along the waves. I pass The Bread Lab, where the day before we had feasted on the most delicious sourdough fresh out of the oven, and then The Old Inn, where fish chowder and mussels had been our treat before a quiz night at Minginish Community Hall.

I'm giggling to myself so much I almost whizz past the point where my van, Summer, is parked in the sunshine and from where I had launched on to Loch Harport an hour or so earlier into the headwind.

It is not the longest of paddles but one I shall treasure especially as it was so unexpected. Leaving Yorkshire for Skye the forecast had not been promising. While much of England basked in a warm March spell, parts of Scotland were being battered by high winds. Pulling over into a lay-by to peek at Eilean Donan Castle, near Dornie, I had nearly been blown over bending down to pick up some discarded litter. The Skye Bridge from Kyle of Lochalsh to Kyleakin had been closed to high-sided vehicles – I gripped Summer's steering wheel holding my breath as we made our way across.

Packing my board and kit had seemed an exercise in optimism over logic when I set off, but it didn't seem right to come all this way empty-handed. I hoped against hope I might get on the water. Thankfully a tiny weather window had appeared on the local forecasting app Marie had shown me and I took the opportunity to launch close to the Talisker Distillery, popping a donation into the Carbost Pier box for parking.

The wind had been stronger than forecast but I was perfectly safe, and my heart is now full.

And as always, I have that unique feeling that only paddleboarding gives me. It is the same feeling I had when I first stepped on a paddleboard on 24 September 2016 in the Lake District – that I am a 'warrior not a worrier'. The revelation all those years ago was especially empowering given worrying has been my default position my entire life.

I am humbled yet strengthened by time on my paddleboard. I am at my most alive and yet my calmest. I feel like everything and anything is possible. The post-paddle energy is when, quite simply, I feel like my favourite self.

Perhaps you do too?

As I pack my kit away, I chat to Steve and Hannah, friends from social media, who with their four dogs are on the island in their van. Hannah later tells me about her own uplifting paddle on Loch a' Chroisg near Achnasheen with friends. 'A stunning and beautiful day,' she says. How fortunate we are!

On my way to meet Marie I look back from the road on to the loch – to have paddled on the water gives me a deeper connection to somewhere new.

Bringing my board had indeed been an act of hope over reason given the forecast. However, I have discovered that wonder, confidence and gratitude are only ever a few moments away once I pop on my buoyancy aid and leash and set forth. If there is a tiny chance of being on the water safely, I will take it.

I hope you will also find this for yourself on your own SUP journey and through the stories I have brought together here. I am so proud to share them with you.

Please do let me know where your paddleboarding takes you, the people you meet and the experiences you have.

I look forward to hearing from you.

INTRODUCTION
JO MOSELEY

Hello and welcome to *Adventures on the Water: The power of paddleboarding to change lives*. I am so glad to see you here. Perhaps you have been given this book by a friend who knows you love paddleboarding, or maybe you are browsing in a gorgeous bookshop wondering if it might be for you. Maybe you have been on the water for a while and are looking for more inspiration and connection. Whatever the reason, I am so thrilled to meet you.

My name is Jo, and I am the author of two best-selling books about beautiful places to paddleboard: *Stand-up Paddleboarding in Great Britain*, published in 2022, and *Stand-up Paddleboarding in the Lake District*, published in 2024, both published by award-winning Vertebrate Publishing. The former was the first guide dedicated only to SUP that covered Great Britain. The latter won the Lakeland Book Awards Zeffirellis Prize for Guides and Places 2025. I'm also the host of *The Joy of SUP – The Paddleboarding Sunshine Podcast* and I have a regular column called 'Paddleboarding for Good' in the UK's top paddleboarding magazine, *SUP Mag UK*. I am a proud ambassador for Cal Major's Seaful charity.

THE GROWTH OF SUP

There is no doubt that paddleboarding has experienced huge growth over the last few years, with many people discovering its benefits during and shortly after the Covid pandemic. Paddle UK (formerly British

Canoeing) is one of SUP's national governing bodies; it has seen its membership grow from 40,000 to a high of over 90,000 members by June 2023, with approximately 50,000 members registering an interest in SUP. According to the Watersports Participation Survey in 2022, almost three million adults canoed, kayaked or paddleboarded at least three times in 2022 and there was a greater interest in SUP across the 380 affiliated clubs. More paddleboarders have been accessing British Canoeing Awarding Body regulated qualifications and awards, with over 25,000 SUP-specific certifications issued. Eighty-five per cent of Paddle UK members classify themselves as recreational paddlers, with the drivers being fun, enjoyment and being close to nature.

With the growth of SUP, an exciting library of literature has developed too, with how-to books, travel guides, memoirs and even our first novel. With the 'where and how' being covered so well, I am very excited to now turn to the 'who and why' of paddleboarding, sharing stories of how this wonderful sport has transformed the lives of so many of us in big and small ways here in Great Britain. When the river is flowing too fast or the winds and waves are too high, I hope that *Adventures on the Water* is the book you will turn to for inspiration, guidance and friendship.

I am honoured to share the inspiring stories from our brilliant guests, ranging from huge, demanding adventures to smaller, gentler outings, from names you might recognise and others who are new to you, both young and old. They will take you round the coast of Great Britain and further afield to the Yukon, the Grand Canyon and the Amazon, invite you to watch basking sharks and dolphins in Scotland, surf Northumbrian waves, celebrate community on the Grand Union Canal and whoosh along white-water in Wales. You will wobble, fall, laugh and cry, feel anxiety, courage and frustration, experience a sense of peace and share their triumphs with them.

We have paddlers who were there at the beginning of SUP in Great Britain many years ago and others who discovered the joy only recently. They each have a unique and special perspective to share which I hope you will love as much as I do. Choosing the twenty-five stories has been a huge privilege, and I know, should my publisher have allowed it, I could have brought you so many more. Another book, perhaps!

As well as sharing their stories, my guests have also kindly answered

INTRODUCTION

four extra questions – their favourite place to paddle, favourite piece of kit, favourite paddling drink or snack and their top SUP tip – plus details of how you can contact them and find out more. This is an excellent extra resource at the back of the book so please pop there and enjoy their wealth of knowledge.

My top tip for those new to SUP or anyone wishing to extend their skills, for example taking on coastal paddling or getting into white-water or racing, is always to take a lesson with a qualified coach or instructor.

For me, that first paddleboarding lesson was on 24 September 2016 on Derwent Water, one of the northern lakes in the Lake District. I was fifty-one years old and recovering from an injured knee after a fall at the beginning of the year. Having found the benefits of being active two years earlier, when I rowed a million metres to fundraise in memory of my mum, I missed not being able to move so freely. I was anxious, snappy and had lost that spark of joy and well-being that exercise had gifted. I walked with my eyes to the ground; I wasn't sleeping well and my perimenopausal symptoms and grief weighed heavily.

As my knee healed, I set myself a challenge called 'Rain or Shine 30' – to spend thirty minutes each day outdoors whatever the weather – which I began on the 1st of September. I had seen many inspiring photos on social media and read that as a full-body, low-impact workout, SUP could help heal my knee. My confidence had been knocked by the fall and my research had shown that paddleboarding could improve my balance and core strength which I was keen to do. So, I booked the afternoon with Bo from Lake District Paddleboarding and travelled up with a mixture of eager anticipation, excitement and nerves.

Quite simply, I fell in love that day.

For the first time in a long while, I felt confident, strong and optimistic. As I said, 'like a warrior not a worrier,' and I couldn't stop smiling and chatting on the journey home. I asked for a paddleboard from my family for Christmas and my fifty-second birthday present that year, and on Boxing Day I set out on to the North Sea with my cherished purchase from SUP North UK.

With just that one afternoon's experience on Derwent Water, I also decided that I wanted to set myself the challenge of paddling from Liverpool to Leeds – a total of 128 miles along the Leeds and Liverpool Canal. I was very naive about what it would entail but it seemed an exciting plan. I knew from my indoor rowing challenge for Macmillan Cancer Support in 2014 that I liked a big goal I could chip away at.

However, when I started telling people about my idea, their response was less than positive. 'That sounds logistically complex, quite boring and, well, too difficult for a woman of your age,' I was told. Remember, I was only in my early fifties.

The Jo of today would have dismissed these remarks and carried on regardless. Paddleboarding has given me, and others whose stories you will read in this book, a core of self-belief that I did not have back then, despite having the resilience to somehow manage the juggle of divorce, loss, flying solo with my sons and looking after my dad who was experiencing his third type of cancer.

Back in 2016 however, I listened to the naysayers, doubted my ability and, somewhat embarrassed, I put the dream away. Not away completely, but in a little drawer in the corner of my mind and soul, peeking at it every so often as my confidence grew and my paddling improved.

In January 2019 something clicked, and I felt it was time to take the dream out of the drawer and bring it back into the sunlight. There were two main reasons. The first was that in the preceding months I had been to too many funerals of friends of my age or younger. Vibrant, interesting, creative women, the kind you admired and felt uplifted by after simply being in their company. They had shown me that life is short and precious and, if we have even the spark of a dream, we need to give ourselves the chance of making it come true. Getting to the start line would be something to be proud of in itself.

The second reason was that my youngest son, Johnny, was in his final year at school and would soon be leaving for university. With his brother Henry embarking upon his Masters, the prospect of being a 'single mum empty nester' was looming. I wanted to show my boys that I would be okay.

I wanted to show myself I would be okay too.

I also decided to add an extra thirty-four miles to the original plan so that it included the Aire & Calder Navigation from Leeds to Goole, thus making the journey into a 162-mile coast-to-coast. I would be fundraising for the 2 Minute Foundation and surf therapy charity The Wave Project, as well as picking up litter.

INTRODUCTION

Three years after being told the challenge was too difficult for someone like me, I set off on a rainy Saturday afternoon in July 2019 from Eldonian Village. Three friends braved the weather to cheer me off.

Eleven days, two tunnels, 101 locks, rain, wind and sunshine, laughter, frustration and tears, paddling into my home town of Skipton under the stars and a lot of litter collected – the adventure changed my life. Arriving in Goole in a thunderstorm that swiftly turned to a rainbow I dropped to my knees on the board and sobbed. My friend Jason Elliott had battled strong winds and rain in February 2019 to be the first person to SUP the route. I had now become the first woman to complete what would soon be officially called the Canal and River Trust Coast to Coast Canoe Trail.

The doubters had been wrong. I wasn't too old, and it certainly was not boring as they had suggested. It had been a remarkable modern day SUP adventure on my doorstep in the North of England along a canal built for a time long gone running through towns, cities, rural villages and country fields.

I am thrilled to say that since then a small but growing number of paddlers have completed the route, namely Gee Jackson, Sara Edgar and Sarah Chisem, Julie Kelly and Lucy Norris, Ant Ing and Chuck Norris, Mel Joe and Michelle Ellison, and Daisy Best, who has kindly shared her story with us (page 122).

A film about my journey, *Brave Enough – A Journey Home to Joy*, was made by award-winning film-maker Frit Tam of Frit Films. We are honoured that it has been screened at prestigious film festivals such as Kendal Mountain Festival, Keswick Mountain Festival, Adventure Uncovered and Shextreme.

In addition to the thrill of finally achieving my goal, facing my fears and helping heal my grief and anxiety, being on my board *Grace* – which I named after the RNLI heroine Grace Darling – has taught me the following incredibly valuable lessons, many of which are also echoed in the personal stories that follow.

We are not too old and it's not too late for our own SUP adventure. However that may look for us and however recently we started our paddleboarding journey. As Millie Mears (page 62) and James Little (page 56) will show us later in the book, we are never too young either!

In my 'Paddleboarding for Good' column in *SUP Mag UK*, I shared the story of a group of Women's Institute members, many in their sixties, seventies and eighties, from Elm Tree and Fairfield WI in Stockton-on-Tees, who went for a lesson on the Tees Barrage. They loved it! On local radio the organiser Christine said, 'I'm excited but nervous. But if you don't give it a go you won't know. These are things I should have done forty years ago but I'm doing them now, so I don't miss out forever.' Maureen, aged seventy-eight, added, 'At this age, anything is possible!'

Adventure is on our doorstep. With so many different bodies of water available to paddleboarders, from city canals to coastal routes, we can find adventure in places much closer to home than people might initially expect. According to the Canal and River Trust, fifty per cent of people in England and Wales live within just eight kilometres of a canal or river, and eight million people live less than one kilometre away. I had lived within just a few kilometres of the Leeds and Liverpool Canal for years and never really explored it before SUP came into my life. The challenge created both a new perspective and a deeper love for where I lived and the areas which I passed through. On my coast-to-coast journey, I slept in my own bed for two nights as the route passed through my then home town of Skipton, yet I felt I was on a grand journey of discovery.

We are braver, stronger and more resilient than we think. SUP not only helps us feel more connected to our values and dreams but can also change the stories we tell ourselves about who we are and what we are capable of, physically, mentally and emotionally. This has a positive ripple effect on other areas of our lives, personally and professionally. So many of the personal stories will attest to this.

Blue spaces can have a very positive impact on our well-being. Whether inland or by the coast, man-made canals or wilder rivers and lakes. My body, mind and spirit are strengthened by being on the water. I am always reminded of my good friend Craig Jackson, SUP Shropshire founder and Operational Fire Officer in the Shropshire Fire and Rescue Service, who says that as soon as he is on the water the stress just seems to float away. This is an example of the Blue Mind Theory coined by the late Wallace J. Nichols in his 2014 book *Blue Mind: How Water Makes You*

INTRODUCTION

Happier, More Connected and Better at What You Do. Blue mind is 'the mildly meditative state people fall into when they are near, in, under or on water.'

According to Nichols, most of us live in a 'Red Mind' or 'Grey Mind' state. The former can be used for good when we harness it for action and achievement. However, it can also lead us to feeling anxious, overstimulated and overwhelmed, which over time can result in many of us feeling burned out and disconnected. The latter is when we feel detached, dissatisfied, numbed and lethargic. In *Blue Mind*, Nichols shares scientific studies, including fMRI scans, showing how proximity to water can lead to decreased stress and anxiety, increased feelings of well-being, and lower breathing and heart rates.

Dr Catherine Kelly, scientist, well-being practitioner and author of *Blue Spaces: How and Why Water Can Make You Feel Better*, also writes about how time by water is an antidote to the stresses of our daily lives. 'Blue spaces help regulate the activity of the brain's amygdala, the anxiety and panic centre, because water allows your attention to drift involuntarily and, therefore, more peacefully, rather than being forced or directed,' she explained in an article for *Top Sante* magazine. 'Blue space is more than a neutral backdrop, though – it's alive not just with its own wildlife and vegetation, but with you and your emotions. It changes the neurological patterns of your brain, leaving you feeling more calm, peaceful and happy.'

Our waterways are interconnected. The discarded crisp packet I picked up in Wigan or Burnley would one day have ended up at the coast. What we do in one place affects not just our immediate surroundings but the wildlife and health of our distant oceans. We can individually and collectively have a negative and hopefully a positive impact on the places that bring us such joy. Caring for the environment is a key theme in the personal stories that follow.

Community plays a huge part in paddleboarding. I was stunned by the kindness of strangers online and on the towpath who wanted to support my challenge and our subsequent film. I simply hadn't expected that anyone would want to join me as I made my way across the country and was amazed when people asked if they could be part of the adventure or opened up their homes to invite us to stay. At the finish point in Goole, teams from Paddle UK (then British Canoeing) and the Canal and River Trust were there to welcome me, banging pots and giving me a big bunch of flowers – despite themselves being drenched in the pouring rain. I had only expected my dad and Frit, the film-maker, to be there. Friendship and support is something that many long-distance paddlers have so fully and joyfully embraced. Adrian Angell, an endurance paddler who has undertaken several huge challenges to raise money for Diabetes UK, wrote in his *SUP Mag UK* article of being cheered on from the riverbank by supporters as he made his way through London on his own coast-to-coast from Portishead Pier on the Severn Estuary to Southend-on-Sea Pier on the Thames Estuary. Sophie Witters and Dave Chant, who became the first pair to paddle from Land's End to John o' Groats, told me about the logistical and well-being support they received from people as they undertook the challenge. If there is an antidote to our tendency to doomscroll on social media, watching people share their joy and friendships on the water is definitely it. 'Bloomscrolling' is at its best after a weekend of sunshine and low winds.

My coast-to-coast really opened my eyes to the roles connection, friendships and community play in SUP. I had almost always paddled alone as I simply didn't know anyone locally who had a paddleboard when I began in 2016. There were far fewer groups online and none where I paddled most regularly at the coast and on the canal. As an introvert I also felt anxious and awkward about reaching out to paddlers I didn't know. With unhappy memories of never feeling good enough in school sports and team games, there was also a lingering fear that I would be judged or unable to 'keep up'.

This could not be further from the truth. As a new sport, we don't have the weight of history about who is and who isn't a 'proper paddleboarder'. As long as safety and well-being are covered, the community is very judgement free and welcoming. We are all still writing the story of SUP in Great Britain and there are so many ways that you can experience it – from a chilled sunset paddle and a picnic to an endurance adventure, the thrill of racing, SUP surfing or white-water, or a mindful SUP yoga or Pilates session, with a group, or alone.

Since those early days, I have come to cherish moments with other people, many of whom I originally met via social media and then had the good fortune to paddle with in person. There is something about moving on the water, side by side, unencumbered by worldly expectations, roles and distractions, that means the conversation flows more easily and often more deeply.

Shortly before submitting the manuscript for this book, I was fortunate enough to be invited to paddle with Arnside Sailing Club, based in Morecambe Bay in Cumbria, after speaking to their club about my books and favourite places to paddle in the Lake District the evening before. It was a dream come true to explore such a unique location. Think fast-flowing tides, the bore, quicksand and shifting channels. Setting out into the headwind, I knew no one and yet within those couple of hours together I had three profoundly touching and meaningful conversations with men and women that I don't think I would have had had we met in a typical social setting. I came away with that same feeling of being a warrior on the water – uplifted, inspired and with a full and grateful heart.

In her book *The Joy of Movement*, Kelly McGonigal talks about the power of synchrony – how moving in unison (as we are when we are paddling together) can help us feel more strongly connected. The research she shared from psychologist Bronwyn Tarr was conducted on strangers dancing together at a silent disco. While music and physical exertion played a role in this 'collective joy', it was the synchrony that was the crucial element. Since reading about synchrony, I have noticed it so often. Next time you are paddling with a friend or group why not see if you are paddling in synchrony?

CAN SUP HELP OUR WELL-BEING?

While I am sure we have anecdotally all experienced that post-SUP happiness, I thought it would be helpful to look at how SUP fits into wider scientific and social research into well-being.

In 2008, the New Economics Foundation researched and created a project called **Five Ways to Well-being**, identifying five key actions that can help us live well. You'll find these outlined on the NHS and GOV.UK websites and by mental health charities such as Mind.

The key actions recommended for Five Ways to Well-being are:

- social relationships and being connected
- physical activity
- awareness
- learning
- giving to others

How can SUP help us with the Five Ways to Well-being?

Social relationships and being connected. We have talked about how SUP offers the opportunity for social relationships and being connected. According to Professor Rose Anne Kenny, author of *Age Proof: The New Science of Living a Longer and Healthier Life,* good quality friendships and family relationships play a key role in health and longevity. Isolation and loneliness are known to cause inflammation, suppress immunity and speed up the ageing process. They are associated with negative physical and mental health, and an increased risk of coronary heart disease, stroke, depression and dementia. In a world where we are so interconnected online, it feels that offline many of us feel more isolated than ever and we are craving that personal connection of being with others 'in the real world'.

SUP is a great way to develop new connections and relationships. As adults this isn't always so easy. Suzanne Patterson, who loves paddling with Dorset SUP in Christchurch and organises sunset and full moon paddles, loves her local SUP community. 'I am always blown away by the number of people who come to these events,' she told me. 'One year we had 284 paddleboarders together at the same time and everyone I spoke to said it was the best experience they had had on the water. This is what SUP is all about to me, bringing people together to live in the moment and enjoy the company of like-minded people. I feel truly blessed and so grateful that I am part of something so wonderful. My mental health has benefitted hugely from paddling. Every paddle feels like therapy.'

Of course, some of us prefer a quieter paddle alone – even here we can benefit from simply saying hello and chatting to people that we might see locally on the way to the beach or lake, or in the cafe we pop to after a paddle. These are what sociology professor Mark Granovetter called 'weak ties' in his influential 1973 paper, 'The strength of weak ties'

– he concluded that they can be very beneficial for our mental well-being. Like the 284 people who went for a sunset paddle in Dorset, we may never go to these people's homes or develop a strong friendship with them, but these casual interactions are important. University of Essex senior lecturer in psychology Gillian Sandstrom also investigated how much happiness people gained from weak ties, noting that on days that a participant had a greater number of casual interactions with weak ties they experienced more happiness and a greater sense of belonging. Maybe that's why so many of us enjoy a paddle with a local group or close to home where we bump into the same dog-walkers or hikers and have a short cheery conversation.

If you are in any doubt, going for a paddle with someone whose company you enjoy is good for you! Mixing the generations is also great for building strong relationships and communities that learn from each other. Anna and James Little (page 56) and Dale and Millie Mears (page 62) are wonderful examples of this.

Physical activity. I am sure we are all aware of the benefits of exercise for our well-being. According to the NHS website, it can reduce our risk of major illnesses such as coronary heart disease, stroke, type 2 diabetes, a number of different types of cancer, falls, hip fracture, osteoarthritis, dementia and Alzheimer's disease, and lower our risk of early death by up to thirty per cent.

Many people say that one of the loveliest aspects of paddleboarding is that they are enjoying it so much it doesn't feel like exercise in the way they have grown up thinking about exercise – something they 'should' do rather than something that might make them feel great. We are having a low-impact, full-body workout improving our balance and core strength without really noticing it. According to researchers from Sheffield Hallam University who did a literature review for Paddle UK, a study from 2016 found participants in a six-week SUP course showed significant improvements in aerobic and anaerobic fitness, along with improvements in core strength and self-rated quality-of-life questionnaires.

According to Kelly McGonigal in *The Joy of Movement*, physical activity has a positive impact both on our brain and our body. For example, she tells us, it impacts brain chemicals that 'give you energy, alleviate worry and help you bond with others. It reduces inflammation in the brain, which over time can protect against depression, anxiety and loneliness.' What I really love from this excellent book is that she shows how regular exercise – let's say paddleboarding here! – 'remodels the physical structure of your brain to make you more receptive to joy and social connection. These neurological changes rival those observed in the most cutting-edge treatments for both depression and addiction. The mind-altering effects of exercise are even embedded in your musculature. During physical activity, muscles secrete hormones into your bloodstream that make your brain more resilient to stress.' Scientists call these proteins that are released myokines or 'hope molecules'. So not only do we feel better after a paddle and more able to face the challenges of life we are juggling, but it also means we are more receptive to joy!

In her book *Move!*, science journalist, author and paddleboarder Caroline Williams researches the links between building core strength, something which SUP helps with, and alleviating stress. 'Any way of moving that activates the core muscles sends a message connected to the adrenal glands via the brain to help regulate stress', writes Williams. 'We don't yet know exactly how, but engaging the core seems to tell the body to calm down.' She also adds that studies have shown that standing up straight brings more positive thoughts. 'Keep your head up and gaze forward for even more benefits.' Isn't that just what we do when paddleboarding?

Awareness, or taking time to notice. Taking time to notice our surroundings on the water is a wonderful way to add to our paddles – paddleboarding offers so many different things to see. I've been fortunate to marvel at snow-capped fells in the Lake District, dolphins and huge barrel jellyfish on the Welsh coast, and starfish in clear waters on a Scottish sunset SUP. Closer to home, I love spotting the old white and black posts marking the distance to Leeds along the canal, the oystercatchers on the beach on a summer's evening or the beauty of a winter sunrise while the rest of the world is asleep.

Katie Owen, whom I met with her seasoned SUP buddy, Fudge the cockapoo, and her friend Gemma Marshall as they paddled the Great Glen Canoe Trail, is a huge fan of making the most of a sunrise SUP. 'Some of my best memories with Fudge are on our local beach, no more

INTRODUCTION

than five minutes from our house. Not paddling very far at all, sitting together on our board as we watch the dawn colours light up the sky before sunrise while enjoying our breakfast. One early June morning, not long after sunrise, we were getting ready to paddle back to shore and head to work when I heard a blowhole puff behind us. I turned round to see three dolphins making their way towards us. They swam under my board and around us for about five minutes before they continued around the bay. I couldn't believe that we had experienced this, together and on our local beach! Fudge was so calm and just sat and watched them with me. I couldn't have dreamed of a more magical time. I am so thankful for our board for allowing us to have these experiences with nature and for seeing places from a new perspective on the water.'

Likewise, Jules Middleton, a Church of England vicar who paddles in Sussex, goes out on the water for peace and space, a chance to simply be in nature. With a very demanding people-centred job, she told me that 'paddling is about connection to something bigger, for me that's a God who created this beautiful world. It's a place to be within and marvel at nature like a demoiselle fly landing on my shoulder, a fish jumping out of the river in front of me, a flash of blue as a kingfisher flits by, that feel like a spiritual connection to the world around me.'

Being mindful and taking notice of what is around us can help us feel more positive, prevent depression and increase our understanding of ourselves.

According to the NHS, 'Paying more attention to the present moment – to your own thoughts and feelings, and to the world around you – can improve your mental well-being. Some people call this awareness "mindfulness" … Mindfulness involves paying attention to what is going on inside and outside ourselves, moment by moment. It's easy to stop noticing the world around us. It's also easy to lose touch with the way our bodies are feeling and to end up living "in our heads" – caught up in our thoughts without stopping to notice how those thoughts are driving our emotions and behaviour … Mindfulness also allows us to become more aware of the stream of thoughts … and start to see their patterns. Gradually we can train ourselves to notice when our thoughts are taking over and realise that thoughts are simply "mental events" that do not have to control us.'

I know I have a tendency to live in the past, ruminating on what

I should have or could have done, or worrying about the future and what might happen. Focusing on the way the sunlight sparkles on the water ahead – the glitter path of joy as I think of it – has often calmed my brain and, like Katie, helped me live fully in the moment and feel more hopeful for the future. I sometimes simply say to myself: 'Breathe in, breathe out. Right now, right here, everything is OK. All will be well.'

Next time you are out on the water, why not take a moment to really notice your surroundings and see what happens?

Learning. Learning something as an adult is excellent for our brain, and learning to paddleboard is something we can approach with optimism and a positive attitude. Unlike a sport we might have been made to participate in at school, paddleboarding can be a fresh start to enjoying the water. Within a short time and with instruction from a professional, many people can soon feel that sense of accomplishment of mastering a new skill. Unlike surfing for example, which has a very steep learning curve, SUP's accessibility means we are soon rewarded. This in turn keeps our curiosity piqued so we want to keep on improving. Research has shown that being curious helps our creativity, has positive benefits at a neurological level, improves memory and patience, as well as creating the dopamine hit normally associated with reward.

With so many different bodies of water there's always something new to discover and study, from understanding the tides and coastal maps, to the heritage of a city canal or how a river is formed. Factor in going from recreational paddling to new skills learned in SUP surfing, racing or endurance challenges, and we can keep our minds growing and improving.

There are lots of ways to keep learning with online courses from Paddle UK, going on a white-water, yoga or coastal SUP weekend, travelling to new places or researching more about the history, culture, fauna and flora of the places you already enjoy. Developing your photography, bird spotting or wild camping skills can also add to your SUP journey.

Giving to others. Research has shown that giving to others, such as simply being kind or volunteering, has many benefits for our own well-being, including: learning new skills, making friends, improving our confidence and self-esteem, building a sense of connection to others,

INTRODUCTION

creating a sense of purpose, keeping our own problems in perspective, gaining a sense of reward and even helping us live longer! It helps counteract the effects of stress, anxiety and anger, and increases positive, relaxed feelings with the release of dopamine.

Litter picking has always been part of my SUP life – fundraising for the 2 Minute Foundation on my coast-to-coast and taking two minutes every day wherever I am to pick up litter or do a beach clean. My personal motto is: *I can't change the world, but I can change the little bit around me.*

Personally, I am a big fan of the 2 Minute Foundation (*www.2minute.org*) and the work of Ghost Fishing UK (*www.ghostfishing.co.uk*).

There are so many ways we can volunteer and give back to our communities and the environment, and paddleboarders have very much taken up the call to make a difference. Along with the causes the contributors have written about, here are a few suggestions:

- Join a Planet Patrol Clean Up – pick up litter and record it on their app or get involved in water testing or a spring or autumn water watch. Founded by world record holder and author Lizzie Carr MBE, Planet Patrol harnesses people power and data collection in its mission to address environmental issues (*www.planetpatrol.co*).
- Be part of Paddle UK's Big Paddle CleanUp (*www.paddleuk.org.uk*).
- Volunteer for the Canal and River Trust on the towpath looking after the canals or as part of their Plastics Challenge (*www.canalrivertrust.org.uk*).
- Support SUP schools and initiatives like Encounter Cornwall's youth initiatives to engage more schoolchildren and teenagers in life on the water with their Ocean School vision (*www.encountercornwall.com*) or Liverpool SUP's Water Wellbeing and Paddle sessions (*www.liverpoolsupco.co.uk*).
- Find out more about the SUP Planet Earth Foundation – this charity works in partnership with Red Equipment to boost teenage mental health by making SUP accessible to young people (*@supplanetearthfoundation*).

- Volunteer as paddleboard support for outdoor swimming events or SUP events (as Simon Hutchinson shares in his story on page 96).
- Become a Marine Medic with British Divers Marine Life Rescue (*www.bdmlr.org.uk*).
- Train to become part of a RNLI crew, volunteer in a local shop or fundraise for the charity (*www.rnli.org*).
- Become a community scientist reporting your plant and animal sightings to iNaturalist (*www.inaturalist.org*).
- Help plant seagrass with Seawilding (*www.seawilding.org*).
- Support the *#PaddleKitHerWay* campaign founded by Sarah Whitney that works with brands to make a more diverse range of kit sizes (*@sarahblues_*).
- Think about opportunities to use your current skills to help others enjoy paddleboarding. For example, SUP instructor Maddy Enoch contacted Paddle UK about using Makaton (similar to British Sign Language) to assist people who may need extra help with communication (*@maddys_sup_world*).
- You could volunteer your skills as a SUP instructor to approach groups who might not be benefitting from paddleboarding. Along these lines, Och Aye Canoe SUP school founder Sarah Thomson works with limbless and sightless veterans to experience freedom on the water (*www.ochayecanoescotland.co.uk*) and Danny Goodridge of SUP Active Yorkshire delivers Paddleability courses training others to deliver inclusive sessions (*www.supactiveyorkshire.com*).
- Become an Ocean Activist with Surfers Against Sewage (*www.sas.org.uk*).

Paddleboarding can fulfil the Five Ways to Well-being in so many different ways. In some areas it is being socially prescribed; for example, Isolation to Inclusion, a Canal and River Trust project, has been successful on the waterways of Leeds. I shared more about this in my 'Paddleboarding for Good' column for *SUP Mag UK*. Funded by Interreg, a European funding body, the project aimed to increase levels of happiness by reducing social isolation and increasing community connection. Using the blue space corridors of the Leeds and Liverpool Canal which travels through the urban communities was key to the success of the project.

Local health data was used to identify people experiencing the highest levels of loneliness and isolation in the communities closest to the canal. Co-creation groups were formed from these target groups. They looked at barriers to participation, what access was needed and activities that could be tried.

Those taking part came to the project after being socially prescribed into local community groups who then signposted them into the Canal and River Trust's offering, which included boating, paddle sports, foraging, bushcraft and poetry writing.

The sessions on and near the water had a huge impact on those attending. At the beginning of sessions, sixty-two per cent of participants said they often or sometimes felt lonely. By the end of the unit, only thirty-five per cent of people felt the same.

One participant said: 'The outdoor activities have given me purpose, hope and brought me inner peace. I've met loads of people in a similar situation to me. It's helped to improve my mental health and well-being. I needed this course to help me on the road to recovery.'

WHAT ABOUT SCIENTIFIC RESEARCH INTO SUP?

As a relatively new sport, SUP has not enjoyed the research attention of other sports such as running, hiking, cycling or wild swimming. However, research is beginning. Paddleboarder and occupational therapist Sara Jayne Kennedy kindly shared her University of Cumbria study 'An exploration of the occupation of stand-up paddleboarding and its impact on mental health and well-being' with me. Participants included a woman called Lorraine who had recently been receiving care in a psychiatric hospital. She said that while she still needs her medication (and of course no one is suggesting paddleboarding is a 'cure all' for mental health conditions or that medication isn't required), she now had another way to manage her condition too. 'There was a point where I stood up ... on the river ... and there was ... green all around me. And I thought this is where I'm going to recover.' Lorraine continued, 'To be able to self-rescue [get back on her board] is by far the most empowering thing I have done for years. I felt like a rock star. I thought, I'm the strongest woman that has ever lived ... and now I teach other women to get back on their boards.'

The research findings concluded that participants experienced enhanced social relationships, reduced stress levels and were better able to manage mental health symptoms.

Sheffield Hallam University's literature review commissioned by Paddle UK into the physical, mental and economic benefits of blue space highlighted that a number of the studies proved the effect to be significant.

Likewise, paddleboard brand Red Equipment conducted a citizen science project into the benefits of SUP with 200 participants over eighteen months in conjunction with Blue Health Coach Lizzi Larbalestier. From the results, Larbalestier concluded that paddleboarding made the paddlers thirty per cent happier, with the top three motivators being:

- enjoying scenery and wildlife
- improving health and taking exercise
- relaxing, unwinding and letting off steam

Let's hope that SUP becomes the focus of more academic research. I will report back when I hear of any!

HOW PADDLEBOARDING CONTINUES TO ENHANCE MY LIFE

I have spoken previously of how SUP changed my life back in 2016 with my first lesson, in 2019 with the coast-to-coast, the launch of my film in 2020, and then in 2022 and 2024 as my first two books were published. If I am honest, I expected that the benefits would now be slightly less significant going forward. A gently upward trajectory of joy and peaceful paddles. I should of course have known better!

While researching and writing this book, I experienced another unexpected plot twist as a long-term relationship ended, I left my lovely job and moved to the coast to look after my ninety-one-year-old father. Starting over at sixty had certainly not been what I anticipated for the beginning of 2025.

However, I feel deeply that being out on my paddleboard, beach cleaning and having the support of SUP friends have all helped me navigate this time more optimistically. Sunrise paddles on the North Sea have reminded me that I am stronger than I think, that I can get back up should I fall, and this is simply another adventure in the winds and waves of change to navigate.

To paraphrase the words of *Little Women* author Louisa May Alcott, 'I am not afraid of storms, for I am learning how to paddle my board.'

Furthermore, it is helping me build new friendships and connections. I was so overjoyed to receive an unexpected WhatsApp message inviting me to paddle at 6.30 a.m. with new friends I could barely sleep. I regularly paddle with friends on the sea where I played as a little girl in the 1970s and I could not be more grateful.

SUP transformed my life for the better back in 2016 and nine years on it is helping me to create this new chapter.

Before I introduce you to the personal stories, I would like to leave you with my personal top tips for making the most of your paddleboarding journey.

- **Be a beginner** – always allow yourself the chance to be a beginner, to start and yes, maybe fall, but to try again and remain curious. Be brave enough to suck at something new.
- **Experience the magic of stepping out of your comfort zone** – every once in a while, do something new: sign up for a group paddle or clean-up, go somewhere you have not been before or go a little further, join a white-water course or SUP yoga session. Why not train to be a SUP coach or instructor to share your skills with others? Feel the thrill of accomplishing something different.
- **Leave room for serendipity** – while it is always vital to plan for safety and well-being on your paddles, leave space in the itinerary where possible for the unexpected. A moment to pause and watch for kingfishers or dolphins, chat to people along the towpath who might share some interesting history or wait until a rainstorm has passed and the rainbow appears across your favourite lake. Be open to possibility and unexpected opportunities.
- **Put yourself in the way of awe and wonder** – if you can, paddle among the mighty fells of the Lake District, experience

SUP in the city, notice the tiny damselflies flitting along the riverbank or the smell of lavender on the towpath, or simply sit with your flask of tea and cake and watch the tide ebb and flow after your paddle. Whether you have a religious or spiritual practice or not, allow yourself to marvel at something bigger beyond our normal, screen-focused days.
- **Surround yourself with people who lift you up** – paddleboarding is full of inspiring role models and people who want you to enjoy the SUP life too. They will add to your joy immensely.

I am so honoured and excited to now introduce you to the wonderful contributors who have generously shared their stories about how SUP has transformed their lives. We all want you to experience the same joy.

Wishing you all the very best in your SUP journey – I hope to one day see you on the water!

PADDLEBOARDING WITH ORCAS
CAL MAJOR

In all my years of being on or in the ocean – in double-overhead waves, gale-force winds, jagged cliffs and currents sweeping me out to sea – I had never felt so vulnerable as I did when in the presence of these incredible creatures. I could also not think of a more beautiful or privileged moment I had shared with an animal or with the sea.

I'm definitely a morning person. I think I might actually be quite an annoying person to be around in the morning. I have a lot of energy and excitement for the day ahead. I'm cheerful, talkative, irritatingly positive and chirpy. I normally get my best work done in the morning, and I train early because that's when I feel strongest and most capable. Evenings on the other hand – imagine the exact opposite, to the point of being almost non-functional. At about 8 p.m. most evenings, a switch seems to go off whereby I am suddenly no use to anyone any more, least of all myself. I'm normally asleep by 9.30 p.m.

Sometimes I can't adhere to this beloved schedule. Such as when the winds are light, or the tides are inconveniently flowing in the right direction for an adventure very late at night. Like, 11 p.m. late.

This was the case one day in June 2021 at a place called Tarbat Ness in the north of Scotland. I'd paddled just over half of Scotland's mainland coastline, having set off from Glasgow several weeks earlier. I was on the edge of the Moray Firth – a big expanse of water just north of Inverness, and I really needed to paddle across that big stretch of water to get to the other side so that I could continue circumnavigating my favourite country in the world.

To say I was tired at this point would be a wild understatement. I wasn't even that chipper in the mornings any more. I had paddled day and night on the tides' terms for weeks to keep chipping away at mile after mile of exposed, rugged and breathtakingly beautiful coastline. The stretch I had feared most – the north coast – felt like a lifetime ago now, but the memory of the strong winds, seasickness, crazy tidal races and committing, unforgiving paddles stuck with me.

Also sticking with me was the memory of the three orcas who had joined me on the west coast. Every unusual movement of water since had put me on edge as I recalled their enormous six-foot-tall, jet-black fins speeding towards me, their unfathomable size and grace and the eye which looked directly up at me from the crystal-clear water as one particularly inquisitive female swam underneath my board, turning on her side as she did so to get a closer look at me. In all my years of being on or in the ocean – in double-overhead waves, gale-force winds, jagged cliffs and currents sweeping me out to sea – I had never felt so vulnerable as I did when in the presence of these incredible creatures. I could also not think of a more beautiful or privileged moment I had shared with an animal or with the sea.

After turning the corner at the eastern end of the north coast after John o' Groats, I had begun paddling south along one of my absolute favourite sections of Scotland's coastline. Mile after mile of seabird cities – cliffs and sea stacks lined with puffins, guillemots, razorbills, fulmars, shags and gulls – deafeningly noisy, with a relentless smell of seabird guano (accumulated faecal excrement of seabirds), which had come to feel like a familiar, homely scent. I love seabirds. I paddled far enough away from their cliffs so as to avoid disturbing them, yet still daily I was joined on the water by rafts of adults and recently fledged chicks on their fishing missions – this never got any less special. This ocean haven felt like a million miles away from the cars and traffic and emails of land-life. The hustle and bustle of the busy noisy birds had a reality to it that instilled calm into me unlike the busyness of our own 'ecosystem'. Hours on end with just the ever-changing ocean, its towering cliffs and its myriad inhabitants brought an unparalleled peace of mind.

That is until I made a harrowing discovery on this very same stretch of coast. I saw something floating about a mile offshore, large and white. I paddled out, and as I got closer the oil on the surface of the water and the stench confirmed my worst fears. It was a dead humpback whale. I roughly measured it based on paddleboard lengths, and concluded that it could not be fully grown – a juvenile, floating belly up, a fulmar picking at its carcass. My partner, James, was with me on his kayak, and we got to work documenting what we'd found. Rope around the tail and fluke, creel pots hanging down into the depths. A young calf, less than a year old, likely drowned from entanglement following an unknown amount of suffering.

I felt an enormous amount of responsibility to communicate what we'd found in a way that might educate and encourage positive change. The purpose of the expedition was to tell the ocean's most pressing stories – to film what's out of sight and out of mind – the incredible underwater world full of kelp forests, brittlestars and flame shells. The humpback felt like the tip of the iceberg, a desperate but important discovery.

So, my exhaustion at 11 p.m. at Tarbat Ness, on the edge of the Moray Firth, felt as deeply emotional as it was physical. A mix of sadness, gratitude, responsibility, determination and fear. Ahead of me lay a fifteen-mile stretch of ocean which I would have to cross overnight due to the tide and wind forecasts, with no get-outs if the conditions changed.

The sunset at the lighthouse at Tarbat Ness was beautiful, and on one of the longest days of the year there was still enough light to see by as I pushed off the slip into the cold sea. Before long, everything was pitch black. I turned my head torch on, but all it served to do was partially illuminate the movement of water around my board and create shadows which I convinced myself more than once were six-foot black fins. I turned the head torch off, for fear of looking down and seeing a kraken (legendary sea monster) emerge from the depths next to me. At one point a sound erupted right behind my board – the blow of a mammal – but it didn't sound like an orca. It must have been a seal ... an orca's favourite food. I willed it to find something more interesting to investigate, away from us! In the pitch black, my curiosity for the creatures I love so much had turned to abject terror as my exhausted mind played tricks with me, convincing me that this ecosystem in the blanket of black was now a threat rather than a place to behold.

Cloud cover meant there was no moon, no stars, just darkness. We navigated using GPS, until after three or four hours we could just about make out some lights on land on the other side of the firth. At 4 a.m., we dragged my board and James's kayak up the slip at Burghead harbour and sunk into a bench, wired and relieved. Having made it through without getting eaten by an orca we laughed at how jumpy I'd been at every sound, every movement, at how I had insisted that James paddle within touching distance of me just in case a monster from the deep had fancied a paddleboarder for its midnight snack. It had taken all the willpower I could muster, plus a hefty chunk of encouragement from James, to push off from the slip at Tarbat Ness that night, and the reward for doing so was an unforgettable experience that James and I will laugh about for years to come, and the sense of an even deeper connection to the ocean and the seals which came to cheer me on miles from shore.

And best of all, when we arrived at Burghead at 4 a.m., we were met by Steve, a whale enthusiast who I'd never even actually met before, but who had helped me identify the female orca who had swum under my paddleboard all those weeks earlier. He arrived with a camping stove, teabags, mugs, bowls and muesli and promptly got to work making us a brew and breakfast. At 4 a.m. The kindness of those whose passion for the ocean I share never fails to amaze me.

Once the adrenaline had subsided, James and I crawled into our sleeping bags on a bench in a park, well aware and quite honestly not caring what we looked like, and slept deeply until the harbour came to life later that morning.

I had one last thing to do that day before we could paddle again. And that was meet some people from the Burghead skiff rowing club. They had kindly offered to take me out on a boat for one of their training sessions. Their excitement, playfulness and joy at being together on the water was infectious. I had never rowed a skiff before; many of them had never paddleboarded, but we all spoke the same language – one of appreciation for just how much that environment meant to us. They spoke about the change they felt after troublesome days at work as soon as their oar dipped into the water, about the connection they felt to the bigger picture when seals swam with them, and about the community they had nurtured through a shared love of the sea.

I feel very grateful to regularly meet people who share this passion for our oceans. Exploring our seas translates to understanding them and caring about them. People will protect what they love, but they can only love what they know. And time and again, once people find that indescribable connection to the water, I see them wanting to share that with others.

In 2020 I founded the charity Seaful to do exactly that – to help others connect with our ocean, understand it and protect it. Many of our volunteers are paddleboarders who feel as grateful as I do for having discovered this way of nurturing connection and community which means so much for their well-being, mental health and their ability to care for our blue spaces. Sharing that through Seaful's Vitamin Sea Project is a really rewarding way to nurture that connection in others too who otherwise might not have had that opportunity, and I hope translates to more advocates for our oceans for years to come. Because just as much as we need to push out from the shore and stand up on the sea, the sea needs us to stand up for it too.

SUP SURF IN THE NORTH
HEATHER PEACOCK

It was so glassy, and my board actually started to hum as it slid sideways across the face of the wave. It was absolute magic. I surfed that wave right into the beach and whooped with joy!

On 7 July 2020, I had one of my most perfect moments in paddlesurfing.

My journey getting to this point in time had taken over thirteen years and on this day in particular the search for a good wave had been frustrating. I'd paddled earlier in the day with a friend up in Northumberland, but it hadn't been great. The wind had messed up the waves, so we just had a bit of a social catch-up and got in regardless.

I have always been a 'let's just get in' kind of paddlesurfer. Some people are very picky, but my journey has been almost all self-taught and there has been a *lot* of trial and error. I realised early on that any time in the water was time learning and experiencing the power and wonder of the ocean. Whether the waves have been ankle high or overhead, through wind, rain and shine and every season, I've got in.

By this point in time, I'd moved from my first board – an 11'6" Naish hardboard – through three other boards to my latest board, a Starboard Pro Surf SUP 8' carbon board. I bought it second-hand, but it was in mint condition, and it radically changed my surf experience. It was more agile and faster than all its predecessors; it had more drive and just felt good under my feet. It was also much lighter making it easier to get 'out back' (beyond the breaking waves) through the white-water at my local beach. This can sometimes be a real battle because you can't duck dive (where a surfer sinks their surfboard underwater so they can dive under the waves) a paddleboard like you can with a surfboard. You have to somehow go over the top of the broken waves and you can spend a lot of time and energy getting pushed back towards the beach if you don't get it right.

On this day, the surf forecast was around four feet. I'd said goodbye to my friend and hung around a bit ... something was niggling at me. The forecast was for the wind to drop right off, and I had it in my mind to just go and see what the conditions were like in Bamburgh, an incredibly beautiful place in Northumberland and home to Bamburgh Castle. The waves are best there on the incoming mid-to-high tide and when I got there the wind had totally dropped off. It was almost eerie. There was no one out, just perfect-looking waves rolling in. I got my kit back on and got in.

By the time I got out back, my heart was racing – I couldn't believe how perfect it was. You could almost not see the waves approaching because they were so clean from the lack of wind. I tried for a few waves and didn't catch them. I was actually a bit nervous. Bamburgh can get quite big (for me!) and quite powerful and I was all alone. I steeled myself. I studied the waves coming in, looked at where they were breaking and found my ideal spot where I then waited for a few sets to pass. Then, I saw a set approaching. I gathered everything I had learned to date into that moment, took a breath and paddled for the wave. My board took off and I was away. It was like I was in slow motion watching the blue-green wave ahead of me and feeling the acceleration under my feet. It was so glassy, and my board actually started to hum as it slid sideways across the face of the wave. It was absolute magic. I surfed that wave right into the beach and whooped with joy! There really is no feeling like it.

My paddlesurfing journey began back in October 2007. I landed on the Hawaiian island of Maui for the first time, having found out I was pregnant eight weeks before. It was meant to be a windsurfing trip, where my husband Chris had been invited to be part of a board test team for *Windsurfing* magazine. I decided that I wasn't going to windsurf because of my early pregnancy, but a few days into our trip, we had met a couple called Mike and Angie.

Mike was part of the test team, and coincidentally a retired Canadian Olympic decathlete. He and Angie were so lovely, and I liked hanging out with them. On this particular day, a girl called Mari had paddled to the place that they were renting and stopped in for a coffee – she asked if anyone wanted to paddle with her. My interest had well and truly been sparked, and I wanted to give it a go. But I was nervous to say yes. I had zero experience, nothing with me for getting in the water and no clue what to expect.

Everyone was very encouraging, and Mike lent me one of his rash vests. It was somewhat oversized, but I was grateful and took the opportunity. Mari looked after me and we headed out to sea on the North Shore of Maui for my very first experience of paddleboarding.

I was instantly hooked, even though I could barely walk for the next two days from the muscles in my legs aching … but I wanted to give it another go.

That trip was my gateway in to paddlesurfing. It was where I caught my very first tiny wave.

A few days later it was another beautiful, sunny day on Maui. Light winds, and light seas. The sea glistened and I travelled with another new friend on a 11'6" Naish SUP surfboard which had been given to the board test team for their 'downtime'. We paddled down the coast to Kanaha Beach. The reef beneath us danced in a rainbow of colour, movement and sea life. I was mesmerised.

As we were coming into our final landing spot, my new friend told me that there might be a few waves. They were tiny but as we paddled in to shore my board caught one, and I just saw the reef below me blur into an aqua blue haze. That was it for me. My first ever wave, surfed on the North Shore of Maui – the Mecca of big wave surfing. There was no going back from there.

When I came back to the UK all I wanted to do was to find a Naish paddleboard and recreate that amazing experience. There was no such thing as paddleboarding where I lived in Tynemouth on the north-east coast of England, and as I learned quite quickly the North Sea is a very different place to the North Shore!

I was so naive back then. I had no idea about surf forecasting, no idea about conditions, no idea about how to manage a board in the surf – especially not a big one like my Naish. I got shouted at by surfers, thrown around by the sea, bashed, bruised and battered by my boards and my mistakes. You can't fight the sea – it will always win.

I persevered, slowly improving and eventually getting to be quite competent. It's taught me so much about myself, and on many occasions it's been my go-to for my mental health, as well as my enjoyment, and it's given me a deep connection with and respect for the water. It's opened my world up to new adventures, new people, new places and opportunities. I've caught waves in places I'd never imagined and put the world to rights journeying up rivers, across lakes and 'out back'.

Over time I have learned how to work with the ebb and flow of the tide, and in 2021 I qualified as a SUP instructor.

I really wanted to help others learn so their journey into enjoying time on the water, no matter where that be, didn't have to take a long time! By this time, I had also become really interested in water safety and first aid. So many people had now taken to paddleboarding with the invention of the iSUP (inflatable SUP) and I had witnessed many people struggling with conditions.

This was really the next phase of my journey. Realising that I loved helping people was big. I continued with my SUP, water safety and first aid qualifications, and worked in numerous local surf and outdoor schools in my spare time teaching stand-up paddleboarding to beginners.

I have found great satisfaction in passing on my knowledge to others and seeing the joy that they felt when they got the hang of standing up, got over their fear of falling in or felt the acceleration of catching a wave for the first time.

In early 2022 I decided that I wanted to do more and to give back to the community where I live. I started to volunteer for our local coast-guard rescue team in Tynemouth – the Tynemouth Volunteer Life Brigade. It's given me an opportunity to do further training in water rescue, rope rescue and search techniques, and advance my medical skills.

In 2024 I attended over seventy-five call-outs and, with support from the team, pulled three people from the water and rescued one person from a cliff. I have also given medical care to many and delivered water safety talks to hundreds. It's been the next extension of my drive to help people, and I get a huge amount of satisfaction from that.

I'm nearly fifty now and still learning. Time in the water is time well spent. It's a part of my soul; a part of my story and I hope that will continue for many years.

PADDLEBOARDING HOME
SHILPA RASAIAH

The biggest memory I have is how this adventure turned into a celebration of community and the kindness of strangers. Old school friends I had not seen for nearly forty-five years came out, colourfully dressed, to walk the towpath under the M25 and later came to my club for a SUP taster lesson.

'Exactly one week to go to #supthegrandunion – I'm definitely feeling nervous and unsure if my body will cope with the challenge. I've never in my entire life done anything like this – so feeling apprehensive but also very supported.' *Extract from my Instagram post, 3 June 2022.*

What on earth possessed me, someone who has never done anything adventurous in her entire life, to take on the challenge to paddle 170 miles, the length of the Grand Union Canal from London to Trent Lock in Nottingham? I hadn't grown up being adventurous. In fact, I only learned to swim in my late forties, so what made me take on this challenge?

I had been a member of the Soar Boating Club for a while, but only kayaked very occasionally. However, during the summer of 2021 the club acquired a couple of paddleboards. On my third attempt I fell totally in love. That feeling of 'walking on water', seeing the reflections of the clouds and the amazing plant life under my board was incredible.

In September 2021, I was selected as a Paddle UK #ShePaddles Ambassador joining a virtual community of inspiring paddle sports women. I represented Paddle UK at Kendal Mountain Festival – alongside my hero Brendon Prince (see page 41); I have been interviewed by the wonderful Cal Major (see page 25) and met Jo Moseley, who have all undertaken inspiring SUP adventures.

Becoming a #ShePaddles Ambassador was pivotal and gave me a *raison d'être* to share my love of the water. The idea of a SUP adventure to inspire other women, especially women of colour, along the journey started to take shape in my head. I was fifty-nine, soon to be sixty, I was in good health, and for the first time in many years had space in my diary.

I decided to 'feel the fear and do it anyway'.

Choosing the route was easy as I had lived near the Grand Union Canal. However, instead of choosing the more popular route to Birmingham, it was really important for me to paddle home to my boat club at Normanton on Soar on the oldest section on the Grand Union Canal. The route weaves through interesting places like Cow Roast, Berkhamsted, Milton Keynes, the historic canal centre at Stoke Bruerne, the winding remote areas of Nether Heyford, and through the heart of Leicester and my hometown of Loughborough. I paddled underneath the M25 and M1, travelled through tunnels such as Blisworth and the famous Foxton Locks.

I had only ever paddled two miles at most so needed to build up my strength and stamina – I was fortunate that Dan Lloyd and Andy Oughton stepped in to help. The first time I went on a long-ish paddle with Andy, I fell in the canal getting off near a bank, and had to change on the side of the canal on a cold wintery day. I never repeated that mistake again.

Finding someone to accompany me for the whole journey proved difficult, as no one was daft enough or had the time to complete the entire adventure. Social media, especially Facebook and Instagram, was invaluable in this. Four amazing women – Belle Yates, Deborah Vogwell, Carys Owen and Niki Truebridge – became part of my virtual team. They were especially supportive when a month before setting off, disaster struck. I injured my back and was bedridden, hardly able to move. After about two weeks of bed rest, strong meds, acupuncture and manipulation, I was able to get up and slowly resume the training. My hubby, Gehan, whom I'm so grateful to, came along on practice paddles to make sure I was safe while rebuilding.

As a result of this injury, I was nervous about my ability to paddle 'up' the Chiltern Hills, which involved sixty-two locks along a stretch of forty-three miles. I considered missing this section out, but Shane Morgan, a good friend at my club, suggested that I might regret this. I put a call out for help via social media, and incredible offers of support came from total strangers to stay at their homes and help with portages – these were my 'water angels'.

While I was already buzzing with the kindness of strangers, a miracle happened. A boater couple, Hilary and Richard Whitby, offered to put me up for two nights on their narrowboat at a particularly remote section of my route. I had always wanted to stay on a narrowboat; I think I actually did a little jig when I heard the news. Their offer gave me such freedom in terms of kit and navigating the flights of locks. They met me halfway at Stoke Bruene and then escorted me all the way back to my boat club.

The whole adventure took on a different perspective. Instead of aiming to complete the paddle as fast as possible, my back injury meant I had to be very mindful about what was possible. I decided to do it at my own pace and take time to enjoy the journey.

Just before the launch however, I seriously began to doubt myself – I was only carried along by the kindness and encouragement of my boat club friends and the support of my sister.

Expecting a fairly low-key discreet launch, the reality of the first day felt like a colourful carnival. About thirty-five older women came out in kayaks and canoes to send me off from the Pirate Castle on Regent's Canal. The Pirate Castle was my chosen charity to fundraise for and they led the procession through Central London, with my family and Shane on board their narrowboat. A photographer from *The Telegraph* and journalist Eleanor Mills also joined us on a glorious sunny morning.

I didn't know where to look, I was simply in awe of the situation, smiling non-stop and so happy to be on my way with my lovely friends, the nervous jitters of the day before all gone.

The biggest memory I have is how this adventure turned into a celebration of community and the kindness of strangers. Old school friends I had not seen for nearly forty-five years came out, colourfully dressed, to walk the towpath under the M25 and later came to my club for a SUP taster lesson. Various friends and family made a special trip to come and encourage me along the journey and some paddled with me for a day.

Earlier on in my planning for this trip, I had heard about an organisation called the Boaters' Christian Fellowship – it was a joy to meet up with them at their annual gathering near Milton Keynes. I spent some time with them eating cake and chatting then, when it was time to leave, they prayed for my adventure which I really welcomed. Also, Lorraine Leckenby of the Friends of the Grand Union Canal came out especially to meet me and we did a little litter pick together.

Paddling through Leicester, we stopped off at Abbey Park to meet my ninety-year-old mum and some of her neighbours. This was such a special moment, as she had never seen me paddleboard before. They brought us a delicious picnic and also fed us little Indian sweet treats called *penda*, which are traditionally served at special occasions.

Before the adventure I had been fearful about my ability to paddle the distance, but by about the third or fourth day I started to really enjoy the routine of 'paddle, eat, sleep and repeat'. I was truly loving every moment of it. The Grand Union Canal is incredible, and it was wonderful to be continuously travelling through it, taking in the sights and sounds of nature, the wildlife and being amused by the narrowboat names. The scenery was constantly changing along the route with lots of different urban and rural environments. The days that were the nicest to paddle were when there was no road noise at all. My memory of the adventure is mainly of glorious sunshine, having lunches on the towpath in the dappled shade of trees and hedgerows, and listening to the birds. Of course, there were a few wet days and some very heavy headwinds to contend with, but mostly it was sunny; in fact, it was too hot sometimes.

As the days went by I found I got stronger, faster and fitter. There was a running joke with my support team that I was paddling off in the distance and they could not keep up with me. This was in part because I had got stronger but also because I was getting comfortable with the amazing board that the wonderful people at the Quroc paddleboard company had sent me to use especially for the adventure.

Over time, I felt more positive about the likelihood that I could actually complete the challenge, and I treated it with serious determination. By the time I reached the Soar Valley villages, I felt like I was nearly home – I was on familiar waters and was really enjoying some solo paddling. My support team all wanted to be there for my final day and travelled miles to join me on the water near Loughborough. Niki totally surprised me by bringing some bright colourful garlands which we placed around each other while knelt on our boards on the canal bank. This was an incredibly touching moment for me as the exchange of garlands is used to commemorate special occasions in Indian culture. She also brought some beautifully embroidered caps with the *SUP the Grand Union* logo on them for the entire support team to wear for the final homecoming paddle. Such kindness!

Hilary and Richard had stayed behind to decorate my escort narrowboat with lots of bunting. Imagine my surprise when I saw her cruising up to Bishop Meadow lock at the edge of Loughborough looking all jolly as if she was going to a party!

What I didn't know was that at the base of the Bishop Meadow lock there was a flotilla of some fifty kayaks, canoes, speedboats and paddleboards all waiting to meet us and escort us 'back home' to my club in Normanton on Soar! Among them were social media friends whom I'd never met, but who had travelled miles to be there for my 'homecoming paddle'. As we paddled past the little chalets that line the river near the boat club, folk gathered outside banging on pots and pans to welcome us home.

My heart was overflowing, and I really didn't know which way to look. As we approached the Soar Boating Club there were crowds of people standing and cheering us on. So many friends, neighbours, paddlers and boaters had come out to welcome us home.

I had been asked to hold back while the other paddlers went forward and a finish line was put across the river for me to go past. It was such a sweet touch.

My support team had somehow managed to corner me and Dave Morris sprayed a massive bottle of champagne over me. There were welcome home banners, a big, delicious cake and the club commodore made a speech to welcome me back. This homecoming party was masterminded by Shane Morgan with the support from my lovely fellow boat club members. I spent the evening in a state of sheer joy, chatting with so many people who had taken time out to be there. It felt surreal to be surrounded by so many folk who really cared; I was buzzing, and it is an occasion that I will never forget.

Apart from the jitters prior to setting off on this adventure, I do believe that for most of the journey I was smiling and incredibly happy. It was great to be physically active outdoors on the water for such long stretches at a time. It helped to me feel fitter and stronger.

Paddleboarding the Grand Union has given me so much confidence to believe in myself and to go out and make things happen. I've discovered that I am happiest when I am outside, especially by or on water. I've gone back to my roots of what I loved doing when I was a child growing up in Africa, and that is my immense love of being outdoors. I've since done lots of longer paddle journeys alone and with others. It's truly been the most transformative thing I've ever done in my life.

CIRCUMNAVIGATING GREAT BRITAIN
BRENDON PRINCE

But beyond the adventure, there's a deeper purpose. I work with coastal communities to help them find their course, whether through tourism, sustainability or a stronger understanding of water safety. Because at the heart of everything I do is one unwavering goal: to put an end to accidental drowning.

Have you ever locked eyes with someone and felt them looking straight through you – searching, pleading – for an answer your body can't give? That raw, desperate look that reaches into your soul, when words are useless.

It's the look of a mother, a husband, a partner, a child – someone who has just lost the person they love. A look that never fades, never softens with time. It stays with you; it wakes you in the night. It meets you across a crowded street, stares back at you from an audience. No one should lose a loved one to accidental drowning; I hope and pray you never have to look into a person's eyes the moment they realise they have.

So, this is my why. The reason behind everything I do. Because if my story brings even the smallest step towards preventing another drowning – if some part of my work makes a difference – then I can sleep. Until tomorrow.

In 2021, I set myself the ultimate task: to paddleboard the entire coastline of Great Britain. Not because the adventure of such a record-breaking journey was calling, but to raise my profile, have a bigger voice for water safety and drowning prevention, and to support Above Water, the charity I had founded. Above Water is a water safety education charity, to give children the knowledge, confidence and power to love water and to embrace its wonder, but also to know how to stay safe and help others. I wasn't new to SUP or the sea; I've been long-distance sea swimming and have enjoyed paddle sports in the ocean surf environment for decades. In fact, being out at sea on a thin piece of foam, fibreglass and epoxy is my happy place. A place I feel safe – more in control, and more knowledgeable about than walking down the high street! Taking on a challenge that others had tried but none have succeeded at seemed a straightforward one for me. In fact, I kicked myself that I hadn't thought of it before.

The plan was simple, on paper at least. Leave Torquay, paddle to Brixham, then keep turning right. One final right turn, after what I estimated would be around ninety days – though in reality it stretched to 141 – and I'd land back on the red sands of home. But, as you can imagine, what looked straightforward on a map was anything but in the real world.

A paddleboard is not the most efficient form of travel on the ocean. It's awesome in every way, but a kayak or, in fact, any other form of marine travel, is more efficient. Standing on a board that half sits in the water means your entire body is a sail; every ripple, breeze, gust of wind or storm has a massive impact on your ability to travel in a desired direction.

On day one of the Long Paddle, the world watched as I set off. Family and friends lined the shore. TV crews, radio hosts and reporters were there to capture the moment – the start of something epic. The April sun shone, but the southwesterly wind had other plans. At twenty to twenty-five miles per hour, it hit me head-on, an invisible wall standing between me and Plymouth.

The objective of day one was to paddle to Plymouth, a paddle I have done on numerous occasions – in both directions – but never into a headwind this strong. After twelve hours of paddling, I'd achieved less than half the desired distance and pulled into Dartmouth. And that was day one. The brutal reality of paddling our coastline: strong currents, big seas, shipping lanes, military bases, harbours, marine life – all forces conspiring to slow me down.

Lying in my sleeping bag that night, I asked myself: *What are you doing?*

But, after that, doubt never took hold. My mission was bigger than the struggle. This journey was about proving what could be achieved, about pushing boundaries while respecting the sea. It was about raising awareness and funds for Above Water. And I would not fail.

By mid-September, after 141 days and thousands of paddle strokes, I made the final right turn home. The beach at Torre Abbey Sands came into view – a vision I had clung to for months. Hundreds of paddlers joined me on the water, thousands more waited on the shore. The roar of celebration was overwhelming. Stepping on to the red sands, I dropped to one knee and gave thanks for something I could never have achieved alone.

I didn't paddle alone.

Will and Harry followed on land, my ground crew keeping me steady from the shore. Lucy and Zoe worked the phones, making sure everything behind the scenes ran smoothly. My wife, Helen, and our children, Kitty, Roo and Jonah, carried me in ways they'll never fully know. And then, of course, there was the big man upstairs, guiding me when the sea felt endless. These incredible people – and so many more – put the *power in my paddle*. And yet, it took months to truly grasp the magnitude of what we had achieved together.

When you take on a challenge like this, you have to ask yourself: *What is your default setting?* After fourteen hours of paddling, when you land on a beach to find fifty strangers waiting – wanting a photo, a chat, a moment of your time – and you know you have less than an hour to eat, rest, and head back out for another five hours, what do you do?

Mine was to smile.

Smiling is a powerful thing. It lifts others. It lifts *you*. It fuels belief when exhaustion sets in. It turns doubt into determination. For the Long Paddle, smiling was my default setting. And it got me through.

I would smile when paddling in huge seas, smile when very large visitors with big teeth wanted to check out my board, smile when caught thirty kilometres offshore in a storm, smile when putting wet and stinking clothes back on at 4 a.m. for another twenty hours of paddling. It was my way of keeping spirits high, of keeping my mind sharp, and my focus unwavering.

When I look back on the Long Paddle, I feel nothing but joy. It was more than just a journey: it was 10,000 stories, eight million paddle strokes and the springboard for everything that has come since.

Paddling is a huge part of my life. With each year, new challenges push my skills, experience and profile further. I organise some of the UK's biggest SUP events, help shape destination development and somehow find myself part of conversations and opportunities I never imagined.

Because when you've paddled every inch of this island's breathtaking coastline, visited every beach and spoken to the people who call them home, people want to talk to you. They want to know how does *their* stretch of coastline compare? What's the best place in Great Britain to paddle? The most beautiful beach? And, of course, what was the scariest moment of all?

But beyond the adventure, there's a deeper purpose. I work with coastal communities to help them find their course, whether through tourism, sustainability or a stronger understanding of water safety. Because at the heart of everything I do is one unwavering goal: to put an end to accidental drowning.

The Long Paddle may have ended, but the tide keeps pulling me forward. And if I get to keep paddling while I do it, even better.

Having circumnavigated Great Britain, I wanted to create more opportunities for others, so I founded SUP Twelve in April 2023 in Torbay. This event runs for twelve hours from 7 a.m. to 7 p.m. with one very simple objective – who can paddle the greatest number of laps of a 3.5-kilometre course in those twelve hours.

SUP Twelve has grown over the years, and in June 2026 we will be bringing the biggest SUP event ever to the UK with the 2026 ICF SUP World CUP: English Riviera. As event director I have huge plans for this event and how the SUP community will be stronger from its impact and legacy. Watch this space and get involved!

This summer, Above Water will impact the lives of 100,000 children, teaching water safety and drowning prevention skills. But living on an island we need to do more. The sad reality is a child will drown this summer because they have never received water safety teaching. Above Water is here to give *every* child these essential life skills.

As for those big questions? Well, you'll just have to ask me sometime ...

SUP YOGA: EMBRACING THE WOBBLE

KATHY MARSTON

SUP yoga gave me a space to process the anxiety, to let go of the past's weight and to find new ways of moving through life with greater presence, fluidity and resilience.

I looked out at the windswept lake with slight trepidation. The water stretched out before me, vast and unpredictable – big, cold and windy. For a seasoned water sports lover, this was nothing out of the ordinary, but for me, a complete beginner in this particular situation, it was overwhelming. The thought of practising yoga on a board in the middle of it all seemed downright ridiculous and well outside my comfort zone. But as Belinda Kirk's *Adventure Revolution* philosophy echoed in my mind – stepping outside the comfort zone is where the magic happens – I gathered my courage.

'Here goes!' I muttered to myself, as I gingerly slid from land to board and paddled out, battling the fierce headwind. I had no clue how to manoeuvre the board against it, and my heart thumped wildly in my chest. I was soaked up to my knees as I focused all my energy on staying upright.

Don't fall in ...

Well, I didn't fall in. But, oh, I felt every muscle in my body working hard to keep me from tipping over. Stand while the water sloshed beneath me? You've got to be kidding! Kneeling was pushing the edges of my comfort zone, and that's exactly where I stayed.

We hooked up to a rope in the water and paused for a moment to take stock. This was definitely not the serene, still-water experience I had envisioned. The wind and waves tossed the board relentlessly, and the only position I could manage without shaking uncontrollably was tabletop.

And then, something unexpected happened. I began to laugh. A deep, earthy laugh that bubbled up from nowhere. How ridiculously fun was this?

I stretched one leg long, tapping my toes to the back of the board, catching myself in a major wobble that almost sent me into the water. Eek! This was liberating. Laughter followed.

I then moved into a wobbly plank, smiling despite the instability, and attempted to lift my hips into what I hoped looked like a downward dog pose. My alignment didn't matter in that moment – it felt strong, and I was rooted in the present. My breath softened, and my brain slowly recognised the familiar motions, easing into this challenging new environment.

A gust of wind sent me crashing back into tabletop, and I couldn't help but chuckle. This was the perfect antidote to the stresses of raising children who had struggled with chronic health issues and hospital stays for the past fifteen years.

Could I stand? I noticed the wind had subsided a little and decided to try. I stretched long into plank, up into downward dog, and began walking my feet toward my hands. As a gust of wind picked up again, I softened into the pose, pausing until the wind passed.

Now this was new. My body was learning to adapt, and fast. I wasn't tightening up any more; my breath no longer showed signs of stress.

When my feet finally met my hands in forward fold, I kept my gaze fixed on the board, not noticing the curious swan that swam by. I was fully in the moment, moving with the natural rhythm of the water beneath me. My heart rate slowed, my mind quietened and a permanent grin spread across my face.

I cautiously lifted one hand from the board, bringing it to my knee – three points of contact on the SUP. I felt the sway and my body's search for that elusive midline. 'Root down to rise,' I whispered to myself, widening my feet to find stability, but keeping it soft.

At that moment, standing up in mountain pose (yogis know it well) seemed to come with minimal effort. The rocking of the board actually felt playful. I was finally in tune with the flow.

That first experience was unforgettable. After the session, I felt lighter and more grounded than ever before. It was as if the combination of water, movement and challenge had unlocked a part of me I'd lost over the years. I'd rediscovered my playful side, the one that had been buried beneath the weight of life's responsibilities. In that moment, I realised how powerful it can be to reconnect with the body, to practise presence and to embrace movement as a form of well-being. The peace that followed – both physical and mental – was a reminder that sometimes, the simplest adventures lead to the deepest healing.

SUP yoga also became an incredible antidote to the built-up stress of my life. Time on the water, surrounded by the open sky, the rustling wind and the waves, was a direct contrast to the sterile, often high-stress environment of hospitals where I spent so many years with my children. The blue mind effect – the calming, healing benefits of being near water – became so apparent to me. Nature has a unique way of resetting the nervous system, and every session on the water felt like a gentle release of tension and emotional baggage.

The more I practised and taught SUP yoga, the more I became aware of how stress and tension held in the body could be linked to specific events or periods of my life. Those deep breaths, the swaying of the board and the unpredictable nature of the water gave me a real-time opportunity to notice where I was holding on. I learned to soften, to release and to respond with ease rather than with the tight, rigid reactions that had served me in crisis but no longer felt necessary. SUP yoga gave me a space to process the anxiety, to let go of the past's weight and to find new ways of moving through life with greater presence, fluidity and resilience.

Yoga balance poses are often associated with finding relative stillness, a reduction of wobbles, ultimately finding that perfect stillness and then declaring ourselves as 'good'. But what if we reframed the idea of being 'good at balance' as being able to respond well to instability? The wobbles themselves become a welcomed feedback loop for each moment of movement. The more we embrace the wobble, the more we become dynamic and fluid, building trust in uncertainty. This wasn't just about balancing on the board – it was a training ground for easeful movement and responsiveness. We learn not to react stiffly to instability and uncertainty, but to flow with it, to adapt and to grow. And what a training ground it could become for real life, where instability and change are inevitable, and how we respond to them is up to us.

These early sessions cemented a huge learning curve, not only about how to navigate this new world of SUP yoga, but how to share it with others. I wanted to be able to help people to experience those same insights into their bodies and minds in just ninety minutes.

In 2018, I took the plunge and decided that juggling family life with my own business was possible. The reality of balancing both was challenging, though. As a mother who had spent years caring for children with chronic health issues, the transition to entrepreneurship felt daunting. Some days, it seemed like I was constantly torn between making sure my family's needs were met and getting my business off the ground. My days started before the sun rose with early morning set-up and ended long after the kids had gone to bed, often with late-night clean-ups after classes.

Paddleboards were purchased, along with an assortment of wetsuits, bobble hats and neoprene leggings, and to my surprise, the classes filled up fast. We had a mix of complete beginners, seasoned paddleboarders and fellow yoga teachers all coming together, cheering each other on.

We tossed out the idea of fashionable gear and dressed for comfort, moving freely in the elements. Whatever it took to stay warm and feel good while moving on the water. And it worked. Our season stretched from mid-April to September without a hitch.

I'd guide my clients for an hour, then we'd transition into 'play'. The class always took a turn when I uttered the word 'now'.

'Now' we'd try poses that felt impossible on a SUP. Tree pose. Hand to big toe. Hula-hooping. You name it, we gave it a shot.

We coined the phrase 'embrace the wobble'. And the more we embraced the wobble, the more confident everyone became. Falling in wasn't something to fear. It became just another part of the fun.

Curious about the effects of SUP yoga, I turned to every book and resource I could find on movement, adventure and well-being. And one book stood out above the rest.

Belinda Kirk's *Adventure Revolution* underscores the power of adventure on our well-being. Could it be that my small offering on a Cotswolds lake could be considered an adventure? After all, these classes were designed to push people out of their comfort zones in a safe, sheltered environment. The challenges, the laughs, the bonding – it was an adventure of its own.

One recent full moon evening SUP yoga session reminded me of the profound power of community. What started as a small class had grown into something much bigger, connecting people not just with yoga, but with each other.

I had a speech ready to share, but when I stood on the board surrounded by yogis, I found myself lost for words. Knowing that friendships had blossomed in these classes, taking people from strangers to kindred spirits, was overwhelming.

'Friendship ... is born at the moment when one man says to another, "What! You too? I thought that no one but myself ... "', wrote C.S. Lewis.

I'll never deny the work that goes into organising and running these SUP yoga sessions. It's immense. But have I ever regretted it? Not once. The struggles of juggling my business with family life are worth it, because I've made friends for life, and I've found a joy I never knew existed.

And I think for me that's what Belinda Kirk's *Adventure Revolution* is all about: not just stepping outside your comfort zone but finding your tribe and embracing the adventure that life offers, no matter how small or big. The challenge of balancing family and business only deepened my gratitude for the chance to bring people together in such a fun, adventurous way. In the process, I found a deeper sense of well-being – a balance between my mind, body and heart – that I carry with me every day.

SUNRISE SUN SALUTATIONS AFTER A STROKE

CATHY MILES

Paddleboarding has brought me so much – a serene sense of calm, a connection to nature, a community like the Paddle Cabin which has a very special place in my heart and with whom I shared that magical sunrise on Bewl Water. I can paddle into the middle of a lake, river or canal and feel untouchable. I SUP with lots of different groups, and everyone accepts me for who I am – a proud stroke survivor with certain physical limitations.

As I sit in the middle of my local reservoir, Bewl Water, I think of how lucky I am to be here. Lucky to be alive. Lucky to be on my paddleboard doing sun salutations, or rather my modified version of sun salutations. It is 8 a.m., the sun is just visible on the horizon as it slowly edges its way upwards. We all marvel at the sight. It is absolutely magical. At one point we are in what I can only describe as a white-out. For about ten minutes we can't see more than a few feet in front of us. It all adds to the mysterious atmosphere. Eventually everything clears and we are in brilliant sunshine.

When Hayley Browning, co-founder of the Paddle Cabin, suggested a sunrise paddle, I immediately signed up. However, I so very nearly turned over to switch the alarm off when it sounded. I literally had to drag myself out of bed. When I arrived, I saw that lots of my friends were already there, so I busied myself getting ready. I take approximately twice as long as everybody else to do so.

My Instagram handle, *@the_disabled_paddler*, may explain why.

In 2017 I was on my third length of a swim fit session when my head imploded, or at least that's what it felt like. It was as if someone had hit me on the back of my head with a crowbar. As I hauled myself out of the pool, I scanned the bottom hoping to see what had hit me so violently. The lifeguard suggested I sit on the side and then later that I move to a room on my own. By now the 'Anvil Chorus' was playing in my head. I knew I had to get to my phone to ask my son, Oscar, to collect me. Dazed and confused I made my way back to the changing room. I threw up several times on the journey home. My husband, Ian, was cooking supper, but I told him I wouldn't be eating as I was going straight to bed.

The next morning, I woke feeling slightly odd, but couldn't quite put my finger on why. I realised my right arm wasn't doing what I thought I was telling it to, well certainly not at an acceptable speed. I asked Ian if he thought I could have had a stroke, and he dismissed the thought immediately. I wasn't so sure. I wasn't experiencing any of the classic FAST symptoms. However, I decided to phone the GP surgery. Unfortunately, I received short shrift from the receptionist when I mentioned that I might have had a stroke and was told I could come along to the surgery if I wished, but the doctor would decide if he had time to see me. She put the phone down but a few minutes later rang back to say the doctor would see me as soon as I could get there.

A CT scan confirmed that I had had a brain haemorrhage inside my skull measuring ten by four centimetres. I was told that the swelling would have to reduce and was discharged with a warning not to fly or drive for six and four weeks respectively.

At home, twenty-four hours later, I decided to have a shower. I'd just put shampoo in my hair, and I felt the same headache returning. I remember contemplating what I should do for the best – should I rinse the shampoo out of my hair or turn off the water and try to get back to my bed? After a few minutes dithering I decided on the latter.

I managed to get halfway across my bedroom floor before I threw up and passed out.

I woke up two-and-a-half weeks later with my skull stapled together and a straw sticking out of my head. I was completely paralysed on my right-hand side.

Ian had found me unconscious on our bedroom floor and called 999. I was taken by air ambulance to King's College Hospital in London and

Ian arrived sometime later by car. The surgeon had waited for him to ask if he wanted them to save me. His reply, which I only found out six months later, was that they should do everything they could to save me, not because he couldn't bear to live without me but because I'm Irish and would only come back to haunt him. Funny and also true – I would have!

I screamed when Ian told me what had happened to me.

I spent a further five weeks on a stroke ward at my local hospital in Tunbridge Wells. I must have twisted my lower back at some point and found sitting for long periods absolutely excruciating. Eventually I got used to being in a wheelchair and enjoyed being outside as it meant my dogs Daphne, a Jack Russell, and Dolly, a long-haired Chihuahua, could come and visit me.

The hospital team recommended a move to a brain injury rehabilitation unit near Ashford, where I would receive physiotherapy, occupational therapy, and speech and language therapy to help with my aphasia, plus hydrotherapy and massage therapy. The chief physiotherapist introduced herself to me within a few hours of my arrival. On the basis that most homes have stairs, she wanted me to climb up a set of steps there and then. It was like someone suggesting I climb Everest. It took forever, but I'm very pleased to say that I achieved the goal and reached the top. I will always be grateful to her for testing me in that way.

I arrived at the brain injury rehabilitation unit in a wheelchair but twelve long weeks later I walked out on my own two legs.

There are a lot of things that people don't discuss about having a stroke – one of which is incontinence as my neural pathways do not let the signal get from my brain to my pelvic floor. There is a big black hole where the pathways used to flow. The good news is I am on a list for surgery, the bad news is no one has any idea when.

The other thing no one is that forthcoming about is post-traumatic stress disorder and high anxiety. I keep seeing the operating staff, dressed in costumes from the *Rocky Horror Show*, dancing and singing as if my brain being opened and exposed is the most normal thing in the world. I also have recurring nightmares relating to my experience in the swimming pool when I thought I'd been hit on the head with a crowbar.

During my recovery, I read a memoir by Fiona Quinn called *Ignore the Fear*. In 2018 Fiona, who was afraid of the sea, became the first woman to paddleboard from Land's End to John o' Groats (LEJOG) on an inflatable paddleboard – a distance of 800 miles.

I'd always been attracted to paddleboarding and thought if Fiona can ignore her fear to paddle the length of the country, then so can I. My first experience was with my two partners in crime, Daphne and Dolly. I signed up for a 'Pups on SUPs' evening paddle at a local lake in September 2020. We had the best time ever – I didn't even get wet. 'How hard could paddleboarding be?' I wondered.

My next experience was in November 2020 – I had a lesson which did not go well and knocked my confidence greatly. Despite this, I didn't want it to be the end of my paddleboarding journey. I had already ordered myself a Red 12'6" Voyager board, having double-checked that that was what Fiona Quinn had successfully completed her LEJOG on.

It would be July 2021 before I got on the water again. I'd found a three-day women-only course not too far away. The instructor had had experience in rehabilitation of brain injured service people, so I felt very comfortable with him.

In 2023 I'd booked a lesson with white-water paddler and Wotbikini SUP school founder, Emma Love, but for one reason or another I didn't feel confident so bailed more than once. We eventually had our lesson, and she was patient and kind. We discovered that I had stiffness in my right leg which was hampering my attempts at standing. I also find it difficult to stand when my right foot insists it wants to be at a forty-five-degree angle, and nothing will shift it. Between us we found a solution together such that if we stacked our bags one on top of each other on the board, I could then climb up to standing. I was ecstatic!

My paddleboarding journey has had lots of ups and downs. In March 2024, having lost my confidence, I had a brilliant lesson with Emily King (see page 112) who had suggested I come to Wales for the #ShePaddles Summer Celebration Festival. I had the most brilliant experience on white-water on an arc, a large rubber ring, where you fly down on your tummy. I was holding on to a volunteer's feet to start with but soon was going solo. Next up was the donut, an inflatable two-person kayak, where I kept forgetting to paddle because of the adrenaline rush! The grin on my face was worthy of any Cheshire cat.

I was also recently invited to the Houses of Parliament for a second time, on this occasion representing Paddle UK at the tenth birthday celebrations of the National Lottery-funded This Girl Can campaign which is focused on encouraging more women and girls to be active in ways that work for them.

Paddleboarding has brought me so much – a serene sense of calm, a connection to nature, a community like the Paddle Cabin which has a very special place in my heart and with whom I shared that magical sunrise on Bewl Water. I can paddle into the middle of a lake, river or canal and feel untouchable. I SUP with lots of different groups, and everyone accepts me for who I am – a proud stroke survivor with certain physical limitations.

I hope to conquer standing on my paddleboard one day and while I know it is a psychological hurdle it doesn't mean it isn't hard to overcome. I'm not even sure what's holding me back as I am definitely not afraid of falling in.

As I say, if you don't try, you'll never know. Watch this space …

MOTHER AND SON RACING TOGETHER
ANNA AND JAMES LITTLE

ANNA

But it wasn't just about competition – it was about family.

It was a breathtaking day in the Lake District. The morning sun cast golden ripples over Windermere as my husband dropped me and my board at the northern tip of the lake, ready to take on the early morning summer solstice race – an eighteen-kilometre stretch down the lake. He also dropped off our son, James, further along the course, so he could paddle the final leg with me.

As the starting horn sounded, a sea of paddleboards and kayaks surged forward, but I had only one goal – reaching James. The first thirteen kilometres flew by in a blur of focus and exhilaration. Speed, rhythm, freedom – I was in my element. Then, in the distance, a small figure appeared, standing tall on a kids' Red race board. James. Side by side, we tackled the final five kilometres, pushing each other forward, revelling in the vastness of the open water and the pure, unfiltered joy of movement. As we crossed the finish line together – first female, first junior – a deep sense of satisfaction and joy washed over me.

My love for paddling began with a good friend on the River Tyne; when I saw Newcastle from the water's perspective I was hooked. The thrill of gliding across the surface, the social camaraderie and the sheer speed of it all which kept me warm! It felt like racing was meant for me.

In 2017, I entered my first paddleboard race. The energy, the people and the sheer encouragement from fellow racers was very welcoming. That summer, we packed up as a family and headed to Llyn Tegid (Bala Lake) in Wales, camping under the stars and competing in the Race the Train SUP event. The more I raced, the deeper my passion grew. My husband and all three boys often joined in, but it was James, my eldest, who developed an unshakable love for all things water. Whatever he tried – SUP, surfing, kitesurfing, foiling – he not only loved but excelled at.

We travelled across the UK, racing in the GBSUP series, and beyond. But it wasn't just about competition – it was about family. Picnics in the middle of the River Tyne with our boards linked together, paddling out to sea, fishing from our boards, towing dinghies and, of course, plenty of jumping in! Staying active and having fun as a family has always been my priority.

After winning the N1SCO GBSUP series in 2018, I set my sights on a new challenge – bringing SUP racing to the North East. So many events were concentrated down south; the miles we had travelled to attend events made me determined to change that.

With Bruce Smith, who trained with us and became like a second dad to James and a training partner to me, we founded the Northern SUP Race Club and the Northern SUP Race Team. With a grant from Sport England and a bit of paperwork, we secured a fleet of N1SCO inflatable race boards and, just like that, the club was born.

Over the years incredible people have passed through our club, not just training but lifting each other up. Watching paddlers conquer their fears, enter their first races and achieve what once seemed impossible is beyond rewarding. Our motto – dream, believe, commit, achieve – couldn't be more fitting.

But I wasn't done yet. While SUP races were growing across the UK, the North East was still underserved. I had to do something. The Beadnell Belta was the first big event I organised: a true ocean tech race, inclusive and exciting, with categories for elite racers, beginners and kids. Soon after, The Big Dippa followed in Whitley Bay, a race born from a collaboration with Mark Ward from Northerly Swell. Live music, food, a bar and thrilling paddleboard races – it became an instant hit. Watching people push their limits outdoors, achieve and, most importantly, enjoy themselves is an indescribable feeling.

I also continued to race. An unforgettable race experience was paddling 100 kilometres across Scotland in under twelve hours on a tandem SUP. The training, the mental grit, the sheer exhilaration of seeing just how far my body could go – it was a day of pure adventure. Loch Ness stretched endlessly before us, its vastness humbling. Every ten kilometres, we rewarded ourselves with peanuts or pork pies – small victories in a massive challenge. Danny Godridge was the ultimate wingman, keeping me motivated and focused.

And then came Florida for the International Canoe Federation (ICF) SUP World Championships. Racing alongside the best in the world was surreal. James, now competing as a top junior, stood beside me as I raced in the over-fifties category. He held my jumper after my warm-ups, carried my board and met me at the finish line with his old mum's shoes! That was special.

I arrived in Florida feeling strong, having trained hard, especially in the gym. My sprinting felt good thanks to hours of training alongside James. In the heats, I finished just one second behind the 2023 World Champion, igniting an unstoppable determination within me. On the final day – after battling through quarters and semis – I shut out every doubt, every distraction. I gave it everything.

Now, I still have to pinch myself. I'm a world champion. But more than that, I hope my journey inspires others – especially older women – to chase their passions, to never let age be a barrier and to keep doing what they love.

Because the water is always waiting. And the adventure never ends.

JAMES

One of the best parts? Sharing it all with my family, especially my mum. Racing together has made it so much easier to travel to events, and we totally get each other – we know when to push, when to help and when to just hand over snacks.

I've been obsessed with the sea and water sports since I was a kid.

There's just something about the waves – the freedom, the thrill, the occasional unexpected dunking – that keeps me coming back for more.

———

It was 7 a.m. and I couldn't even see the sea. The mist was so thick it felt like I'd woken up inside a cloud. But I knew that this was going to be an epic day.

My mission? Set up a safe but challenging course for the Beadnell Belta. As we zigzagged around in the safety boat, dropping buoys into the sea at the right distances, my excitement grew. The swell was big. Really big. And I love that.

The race started a little late because we had to actually see where we were paddling first. Once the mist lifted, I was off, determined to fly around the course as fast as possible. And then came the highlight of my day: catching a wave off the buoy turn and literally surfing past people, what a ride! This was a real ocean tech race, and I hope there will be plenty more like it.

I live for catching waves on my paddleboard or foil board. There's something magical about sitting on the peak of a wave – this perfect blend of peace and adrenaline, along with the slight fear that I might faceplant at any moment. I dream about it a lot.

———

I've upgraded my paddleboards over the years like someone slowly levelling up in a video game. Here's the evolution of my boards (aka my paddleboarding glow-up):

- I started with a junior inflatable Red board (10'6 x 24"); it was good for my step-back turning progress, but not exactly lightning-fast.
- I moved on to a Starboard All Star carbon board (12'6" x 25"), feeling pretty pro.
- I then got a super-narrow Loco carbon board (14' x 19"); balance became very important.

- Today, I use a SIC RS 14.0 carbon board (14′ x 21.5″) – it's fast, sleek and absolutely beautiful.

Every paddleboard race has its own memories. Some are inspiring, some are hilarious and some are … slightly annoying.

One of my favourite events was the SUP Club Championships at Bray Lake. The Northern SUP Race Team finished second but, honestly, half the fun was the road trip. We laughed so much on the drive down and in the hotel – it was basically a team-building exercise with paddles.

Then there was the Battle of the Thames, where Claire Watson-Armstrong was my honorary race chaperone because I was too young to compete alone (thanks, Claire). Fast-forward a few years, and I returned to that race, winning the N1SCO category by overtaking someone on the final buoy turn.

Ah, but let's talk about the Paddle Skedaddle, a twenty-seven-kilometre race I did when I was sixteen. It was going great and I came in fourth overall, but I was disqualified for going round corners too close to the edge (racing!). Was it fair? Debatable. Was the guy who reported me just bitter that I'd beaten him? Very likely.

Competing internationally has been a whole new challenge, but also an amazing experience. I've made friends from all over the world, and racing against the best has given me a fresh perspective and new goals. It's pretty cool to see other young paddlers pushing boundaries, and even cooler to be right there with them.

One of the best parts? Sharing it all with my family, especially my mum. Racing together has made it so much easier to travel to events, and we totally get each other – we know when to push, when to help and when to just hand over snacks. She used to beat me. But now? Let's just say … not a chance, Mum.

Now that I can drive, life has changed. My board goes on the roof, and suddenly, I have the freedom to go anywhere, anytime. Well ... as long as I can afford it. It turns out that adventures cost money, so I work hard to fund my paddleboarding addiction.

My first major solo road trip was to Düsseldorf for the Euro Tour Indoor Sprint Championships when I was eighteen; I competed in the men's elite category. Just me, my car and a long drive through five different countries. Figuring out logistics, driving on the wrong side of the road and navigating unfamiliar cities was a bit of a baptism by fire, but it was totally worth it.

On the water, there are no rules. No two days are the same. One day, it's all about smooth, powerful strokes. The next, it's full-on chaos with wind, waves and the thrill of speed. Every time I get on my board, it's a blank canvas ready to be painted with adventure, excitement and the occasional accidental swim.

And honestly? I wouldn't have it any other way.

FATHER AND DAUGHTER ON THE WATER

DALE MEARS

And there, right beside me, is my five-year-old daughter, paddling on her own. It's a moment I'll never forget. A truly special moment. Perhaps the only thing that could top it is the thought of all three of my girls paddling beside me one day.

May 2024. A loud knock on the door. The delivery driver stands there, holding a cardboard box. My daughter, Millie, then just five years old, dashes full pelt through the house, her eyes wide with anticipation. 'Is it here?' she asks, barely able to contain her excitement. 'Yes,' I reply, and the sheer joy on her face says it all. Looking back, I honestly don't know who was smiling more – her or me.

But to fully appreciate that moment, we need to rewind to 2017, when a similar smile spread across my own face as my first inflatable stand-up paddleboard landed on my doorstep. It was a pivotal moment, the start of a new chapter in my lifelong passion for water sports.

LIFE ON THE WATER

I've been around water sports for as long as I can remember. My dad, a former windsurfer, introduced me to the water at an early age. Many of my childhood weekends were spent at the lake, where we'd take our windsurfing boards out and make the most of whatever conditions the British weather threw at us.

Later, during my Duke of Edinburgh's Award, I discovered kayaking.

It was the most affordable activity on offer – just fifty pence per session at the local lake! You'd never get that sort of deal today. But back then, it was the perfect way to get out on the water, and I was hooked.

Fast-forward a few years, and I found myself at Nottingham Trent University, where I joined the canoe club. With a bit more freedom and the ability to travel, I threw myself into the sport, paddling across the UK and beyond. I was lucky enough to become part of the European Wavesports Kayak Team, which opened up even more opportunities for adventure. Around this time, I also started documenting my experiences online – back when blogs were in their infancy and social media influencers weren't really a thing. Kayaking gave me a sense of freedom like no other. I made lifelong friends, many of whom I still paddle with today.

Sadly, one tragic event changed everything. A close friend was lost to the river, a devastating moment that made me reassess my relationship with kayaking. I realised that my love for the sport wasn't just about me any more – I had a family who worried about my safety. That was the moment I started looking for a different way to stay on the water, and so began my journey into stand-up paddleboarding.

DEVELOPING A NEW PASSION – FROM KAYAK TO SUP

By 2017, SUP was already growing in the UK, but what I saw on social media didn't quite match my own experiences. Instagram was full of idyllic images from tropical locations – paddleboarders in bikinis gliding across crystal-clear waters. But in the UK, SUP looked a little different. There were no palm trees, no golden sands, and certainly no board shorts in the middle of a British winter.

That's when the idea for Stand Up Paddle UK was born. I didn't just want to paddle, I wanted to document what SUP looked like here in the UK, in real, everyday conditions. I wanted to create a space where people could share their experiences, find inspiration and be part of a community.

What started as a simple Instagram page quickly grew into something much bigger. Today, Stand Up Paddle UK remains one of the largest SUP communities in the UK, offering reviews, features and a space for paddlers to showcase their adventures. Alongside Darren Farrar, I've had the opportunity to collaborate with major brands, work with paddle providers and even speak in Parliament about SUP safety, advocating for quick-release belts.

But beyond the events, collaborations and opportunities, the most rewarding part of this journey has been the people. Over the years, I've met countless paddlers – some I've featured on Stand Up Paddle UK, others I've met at shows, and many who have become friends. SUP is, at its core, a community, and it's growing every day.

PADDLING AS A FAMILY

In 2018, everything changed again when my first daughter, Millie, was born. From the moment she arrived, I knew I wanted to introduce her to the water just as my dad had done for me. Sharing my love of SUP with my children was something I was determined to do.

Millie was on a board from an early age, and we've had countless adventures together. Whether it's catching small waves, looking for fish, spotting wildlife or just playing games, some of our happiest moments have been on the water. Anyone who follows my journey will know that she went on to become FatStick Boards' youngest ambassador – a title she wears with pride.

As Millie grew, so did our family. Mabel arrived next, and then in 2023, little Lottie completed the trio. Last summer, for the first time, I had all three of my daughters on the water with me. I can't even begin to describe how proud that made me feel.

Paddling with kids is an adventure in itself. It's not just about getting on the board, it's about the places you explore, the wildlife you see and the memories you make together. One of our favourite spots is Llyn Padarn, a stunning lake in North Wales. The scenery is breathtaking, and for kids, it feels like stepping into a magical world.

Another great spot is Leasowe Beach on the Wirral. The shallow waters stretch out for what seems like miles, perfect for little ones to paddle safely (though if the tide is out, be prepared for a bit of a walk). And then there's Runswick Bay in North Yorkshire, one of Jo's favourite spots. We've spent days there playing on the beach, spotting jellyfish, diving into the sea and exploring the coastline.

But no matter how many incredible places we visit, our local spot at Spring Lakes in Derbyshire will always be special. Spring-fed lakes, open all year-round, offering space to escape and enjoy a moment of peace, whether alone or with family.

A SPECIAL MOMENT ON THE WATER

And so, back to that knock on the door.

Millie, beyond excited, rips open the box to reveal her very own stand-up paddleboard. I've never seen someone inflate a board so quickly! She plays on it in the house for ages, but the real test comes at the weekend when we finally take it to the lake.

We arrive, pump up the boards and get ready. Even though Millie has been on boards before, they've always been adult sized. This time, on a board designed for her, everything changes. We stay in the shallows at first, getting used to the feel of it. Then, after some practice, she stands up and starts paddling.

For a five-year-old, going in a straight line on a SUP isn't as easy as it sounds. But she does amazingly well. Before long, she's following me across the lake, paddling independently.

I take a moment to soak it all in: the stillness of the water, the distant calls of birds, the occasional ripple from open-water swimmers gliding by. And there, right beside me, is my daughter, paddling on her own.

It's a moment I'll never forget. A truly special moment. Perhaps the only thing that could top it is the thought of all three of my girls paddling beside me one day. I know the odds may not be in my favour of them all wanting to come!

For me, that's what SUP is all about, not just the activity, not just the adventures, but the connections we build along the way. Whether it's with family, friends or the wider SUP community, there's nothing quite like sharing time on the water.

NORTH OF ORDINARY: YUKON 1000

SCOTT 'SKIP' INNES AND CRAIG SAWYER

There were of course moments when it all felt impossible, moments when we questioned our ability to continue, but our trust in each other, our preparation and our shared sense of purpose kept us moving forward.

We first discovered the Yukon 1000 in the summer of 2019. A casual search online for a multi-day SUP adventure escalated into a submission to be considered for the 2020 race. While we were both competent paddlers, having been involved with SUP for many years, neither of us had any real ultra-endurance experience. So, on the face of it, a 1,000-mile race that had to be completed within a ten-day cut-off was something almost as inconceivable as the chances we would be selected as one of the thirty teams from thousands of applicants. But in August 2019, we found ourselves staring at an email with the simplest of subject lines: 'Yukon 1000 application – accepted'.

No one starts a journey like this as the finished article – and with the start only a matter of months away in the summer of 2020, we both committed relentlessly to the preparation, training, upskilling and cross-skilling needed to stand a chance of keeping each other alive and making it to the finish line.

In only a few months everything started to fall into place, and we really started to believe that we might just be able to pull this off. But no sooner had we started dreaming of what it would be like to cross the finish line, the arrival of a worldwide pandemic changed everything.

Understandably, the race was postponed. Twice.

The two postponements in 2020 and then again in 2021 meant that what was originally meant to be a single-year adventure had transformed into a three-year journey. But these delays had ended up working in our favour. They gave us time to refine our knowledge, improve our gear and continue to develop our mental resilience. In those pandemic years we learned more about ourselves and what we were about to undertake than we could ever have imagined.

In July 2022 we finally made it to the start line in Whitehorse, Canada, almost three years after applying for the race. But fate hadn't quite finished with us and dealt the cruellest of hands with Craig contracting Covid-19 two days before the race started. With the risks to Craig's health, the possibility that Skip could catch it and the potential spread of the virus to the small communities along the river, it became clear that we couldn't start the race. It was not a choice, but rather a necessity.

The disappointment was heavy. Craig knew instantly that he would return to have another go, but it took Skip a few weeks to come to terms with the disappointment. Skip came close to pulling out completely, but he realised the importance of setting an example to his children that even when the going gets tough, the true meaning of grit is pushing through.

The pain of having to walk away in 2022 only made our return in 2023 that much more meaningful. The training, the patience and the uncertainty over the past four years had made us stronger than ever in mind and body – preparing us to push forward and embrace the unknown.

On 14 July 2023 we left the start line in Whitehorse and our 1,000-mile odyssey was on! The Yukon River is unlike any other river we had ever experienced. The sheer size and remoteness, the unpredictability of the weather, the constant presence of wildlife unaccustomed to seeing humans, and the movement and behaviour of the water made it a survival challenge as much as a race. We faced everything from extreme heat to freezing temperatures, howling wind, driving rain, and the very real threat of forest fires. The water in the river was freezing, which added an extra layer of danger, but we kept paddling. We pushed through, relying on each other, understanding that our only lifeline was the strength of us as a team.

Teamwork was everything. We spent eighteen hours a day paddling in the land of the midnight sun, facing all kinds of challenges. With no outside support and no guarantee of making the 1,000 miles in the required ten-day window, we knew that every moment counted. If we didn't make the cut-off, there would be no extraction team to get us out at the end, and we wouldn't be recognised as completing or competing in the race. That pressure was immense, but we never let it break us; we gave it everything we had. The Yukon is relentless, and its beauty hides its dangers – the wildlife, remoteness and the isolation were constant reminders that disaster was only a paddle stroke away.

As it is an unsupported race it meant there were no checkpoints, safety teams or outside assistance unless things went very wrong and you needed to be extracted. The responsibility falls entirely on you and your teammate to either get through or get out.

The race was not just a test of physical endurance, but of mental resilience and teamwork. It's a race where you learn as much about yourself as you do about the natural world around you. We faced challenges we couldn't have anticipated, but we learned that even in the most difficult moments, it's the willingness to keep going, to keep paddling, that matters. And the beauty of the Yukon, its vast wilderness, and the freedom that comes with being out there, away from everything, was worth every moment of the four years of effort.

There were of course moments when it all felt impossible, moments when we questioned our ability to continue, but our trust in each other, our preparation and our shared sense of purpose kept us moving forward.

We crossed the finish line in eight days, thirteen hours and three minutes and became the first Brits ever to complete the challenge on paddleboards, and were the first SUP team to reach the finish line. For us, this race was never about winning; it was about the journey, the adventure and the lessons we learned along the way. We knew that completing the race would be the real victory.

We are two middle-aged fathers from the south of England, with, at the time of entering the race in 2019, very little survival or endurance experience. If we can do this, it proves that anyone can take on a challenge if they're willing to work hard, learn from their mistakes, grow from disappointment and support each other along the way.

Whether it's the Yukon 1000 or a much smaller adventure, stand-up paddleboarding is an incredible way to explore places few people get to see. And it's achievable for anyone who puts their mind to it.

We hope that our adventure of a lifetime serves as a reminder that there is no dream too big if you approach it with dedication, perseverance and the understanding that the real reward lies in the journey itself. The Yukon 1000 was the challenge of a lifetime, and though we've crossed the finish line, and the adventure is over, the lessons and memories will stay with us forever.

ANYTHING IS POSSIBLE ON A PADDLEBOARD

CAROLINE DAWSON

After five days of what can only be described as one of the most feral and toughest experiences, both paddling and wild camping, we had ever faced on paddleboards, the finish line was finally in sight. The emotions surged within me, and I couldn't hold back the tears. As soon as I stepped on to the sand, an overwhelming wave of achievement washed over me. We had done it.

I found myself craving something extraordinary. I wasn't looking for just any paddle adventure. I wanted one that would create a lifetime of stories and push the limits of what could be achieved on a paddleboard. With the skills, knowledge and determination to take on something remarkable, I set my sights on a new environment – one I had never paddled in before. The Amazon rainforest felt like the perfect challenge. That's when the Amazon Challenge appeared on my radar – a five-day, 337-kilometre paddle down the Madre de Dios, a high-volume, grade-3 river. It was exactly the kind of adventure I was after. The challenge had only been completed on a paddleboard for the first time in 2023. I was determined to be the first woman to take it on.

I knew the physical demands would be immense – paddling for eight-plus hours a day, for five days, in 35 °C heat, while carrying all my gear. It was no small feat. So, in September 2023, Team SUP Lass Paddle Adventures (me, my partner Jon and our friend Matt, who is based in New Zealand) began our training. Most of my and Jon's training took place on our local river, the River Dee, which was perfect for building both endurance and technical skills. The river offers long stretches – forty to fifty kilometres – ideal for endurance training, along with more challenging and technical white-water sections. We did most of our training on fourteen-foot McConks inflatable touring boards, the same boards we would be using for the challenge.

With our fully loaded boards packed with gear, we practised everything – from navigating the river's winding turns to flips and self-rescue techniques. The training was intense, but each session brought us closer to being ready for the Amazon. To gauge our progress and fitness, we also threw in other challenges and races.

Everything was going smoothly until, out of nowhere, I fractured my ankle while on a downriver trip on the Vjosa in Albania (another one of my infamous trips, each with its own set of stories). It was a major blow.

But I quickly took stock and refocused. Mentally, I knew I still had time to recover and get back to full strength. I just had to find alternative ways to stay strong and focused. So, our river sessions shifted to daily gym workouts, and we spent the next two months working on rehab. Little did we know, that wasn't the only setback we'd face …

My first outing after the injury was to join Anthony Ing and Chuck Norris on their Liverpool to Goole charity paddle. I was a bit rusty after two months off, but deep down, I knew I still had the Amazon Challenge in me. Getting back on my board felt like a huge step, and I was determined to start building up my mileage again.

Alongside the paddling, securing support for our trip became another major focus. We were encouraged to raise funds for the local communities we would be paddling through, which meant countless hours spent on social media campaigns and conversations with a wide range of companies.

On top of that, we had to purchase, test and trial every bit of kit we'd need for the expedition. From freeze-dried meals to our poop trowels, everything had to be carefully chosen based on size, weight and how it would be carried. We would be flying out with it all, so there was no room for error. It was a massive logistical challenge shipping five paddleboard bags full of kit and six paddles halfway across the world, but every step was crucial in preparing for the expedition ahead.

By early May, everything was starting to come together for us. We were back on the water regularly, I was fully fit again, and we had completed both the SUP Twelve and the Spey Challenge, even landing on the podium. I knew I was ready.

But then, on my drive back from the Spey Challenge, I began to feel unwell. Over the next few days, my condition worsened, and I was rushed to the hospital with biliary sepsis, requiring emergency surgery to remove my gallbladder. It was a huge blow and couldn't have come at a worse time. I remember sitting in the hospital bed, teary-eyed, telling my consultant that I was due to fly to Peru with my team in three weeks. I was determined to be the first woman to descend the Madre de Dios on a paddleboard. I could see by the look in his eyes that he thought it was a bit of a pipe dream, and that I needed to give myself time to recover.

He signed me off work and told me not to drive or lift anything heavy. It was a massive blow, especially since I still needed to do all those things. My first thoughts were of my team – letting Jon and Matt down, along with our supporters and sponsors. It was a crushing moment, but I refused to give up. So, I went back to the drawing board. I knew I had to make the Amazon Challenge happen. I allowed myself one week of being kind to myself, then I was back in the gym, stitches still in place, working on all the parts of me that didn't hurt. I didn't tell Matt about the setback, as I knew how much he was looking forward to the expedition. Jon did everything he could to keep my spirits up because he knew how much it meant to me.

And so, we carried on. We packed up our gear, managed to find insurance that would cover me post-surgery, and off to Peru we flew. I was anxious, knowing I hadn't stood on a paddleboard in nearly a month by the time we reached the start line. As I stood there, I felt a deep mix of apprehension and determination. I had made it this far. The biggest rapids of the whole five-day journey were less than half a kilometre from the start line, and I was about to face them head-on.

We tackled the first rapid, and the waves were enormous – easily the biggest, highest-volume graded section I'd ever navigated on a paddleboard. Everything was going smoothly until the third wave hit, flipping me completely and sending me tumbling into the water with almost forty kilograms of gear. I stayed calm, quickly flipped my board back over and climbed back on. The Madre de Dios had unleashed her first wild blow, but after that swim, I knew I was ready for the rest of the journey. My focus shifted, and with 336.6 kilometres left to paddle, I knew the finish line was within reach – it was completely doable.

As a team, we worked tirelessly together – leading sections, motivating each other, reminding one another to eat and drink and diving into wild conversation tangents. Over the five days, we even came up with a song, and by the end of each thirty-kilometre stretch, we'd be singing it with full enthusiasm, turning every milestone into a mini celebration.

But it wasn't all easy. The paddle was tough. The heat and humidity were relentless, with little shade in the centre of the river. Temperatures regularly topped the mid-thirties in the middle of the day. We were each drinking over six litres of electrolytes and water per day, and the conditions were utterly energy-zapping.

On top of the physical challenge, we had to navigate through some serious dangers. Our journey took us through areas where there was cocaine production and illegal gold mining operations, and near one of the last uncontacted tribes – the infamous Mashco Piro. We also had to stay on the lookout for some pretty gnarly critters, like bullet ants and wandering spiders. Everything in the Amazon was like a supersized version of what we were used to in the Dee Valley! Fortunately, we were extremely well prepared and carried all the gear needed to handle any emergency situation that came our way ... and for once nothing did.

After five days of what can only be described as one of the most feral and toughest experiences, both paddling and wild camping, we had ever faced on paddleboards, the finish line was finally in sight. The emotions surged within me, and I couldn't hold back the tears. As soon as I stepped on to the sand, an overwhelming wave of achievement washed over me. We had done it. We had completed the Amazon Challenge – 337 kilometres, 58,322 paddle strokes, over 18,000 calories burned, an average speed of 8.3 kilometres per hour, and forty hours, twenty-four minutes and eight seconds of paddling time.

At the end of the journey, Jon turned to me and said my determination was unlike anything he had ever witnessed before. He and Matt had talked about where I had found that inner strength, especially during moments when they had struggled to keep pace with me. I was a woman on a mission, and nothing was going to stop me. It was like a red rag to a bull – the mighty Madre de Dios river was going to be conquered, no matter what.

THE EARLY DAYS
JOHN HIBBARD

Everyone I took paddling loved it, especially the journeying aspect. Even my most die-hard ocean-loving friends admitted there was something special about it. Better still, unlike windsurfing or surfing – where teaching a beginner often meant sacrificing your own session – SUP allowed everyone to enjoy it together, instantly.

I dropped the board into the water and jumped on. By this point in my life, standing on a floating board felt as natural as walking. I was in my element, my domain, my happy place. The only difference with this board was that it was propelled by a paddle, not a sail. It was 2007, and I was a full-time professional windsurfer, just six months away from achieving my long-term goal of becoming British champion. I had barely seen anyone else use a paddleboard – just a few images online – and this was only my third time using one. My first two sessions had been a couple of weeks earlier on the north coast of Cornwall, catching small springtime waves. Those sessions sparked an idea. Not only was there something to this concept of standing on a board with a paddle, but I felt a business opportunity brewing. I'd lined up a third session with a plan to move things forward ... Little did I know that my entrepreneurial dreams were about to come crashing down.

It was a warm evening in May 2007, the sea was glassy, still and utterly devoid of waves. I had convinced Dave Hackford from Tushingham Sails – one of my sponsors – to come down to Bigbury Beach and try out one of the boards. Dave had lent me the board for my Cornwall trip after receiving it from Svein Rasmussen, the founder of Starboard, my windsurf board sponsor, who had sent us a message: 'Stand-up paddling is going to be the next big thing.'

I had called Dave after my first paddle session, buzzing with excitement. Now I needed him to feel that same spark as I did, as I needed his help to launch my plans. Without waves we paddled out 200 metres, turned around and paddled back. We did this two, maybe three times. The novelty wore off fast. It was nothing like my first sessions in Cornwall, where I had been gliding effortlessly on the waves, and nothing like the feeling we got when we did the same 200 metres on our windsurf boards – no speed, no dynamic action. Dave looked at me. I looked at him. The realisation hit us both – this wasn't going to work. If paddleboarding was only fun in surf, its appeal was going to be limited. Surf beaches were already crowded, and surf rage – which incorporates territorial aggression towards new craft – was an issue. If paddleboarding couldn't be fun without waves, then I was seriously doubting the commercial potential.

Disappointment sat heavy on my shoulders. My windsurfing career wouldn't last forever, and I needed something new, something to build my future around. I had dreamed of turning SUP into my next chapter, and within ten minutes that dream seemed crushed.

Desperate to keep Dave's interest, my gaze drifted towards the river mouth at Bigbury. The tide was coming in, and the water was flowing inland. As a windsurfer or surfer, you only end up in the river mouth when something has gone wrong – either you have broken your gear or been washed in by big waves. But today, with no wind or surf, it actually looked inviting. In what can only be described as a lightbulb moment, I suggested we paddle into the river and explore.

Talk about a roller-coaster of emotions – I went from thinking my dream was dead to coming up with an entirely new plan within half an hour. As we paddled up the river, everything shifted. SUP wasn't just about waves; it was about adventure. It was about the journey. Like cycling, where the real joy comes from the ride rather than just pedalling round a car park, stand-up paddleboarding offered a new way to explore. As we paddled under overhanging trees and around bends of the river, the warm evening air drifting past, I realised I was seeing my local waters in a way I never had before. We reached the Fisherman's Rest pub, stopped for a pint, and then let the outgoing tide carry us back. By the time I strapped the board on to my van (it was too big to fit inside), my mind was made up – stand-up paddleboarding was a thing, and I was already writing my business plan in my head. More than that though, I had just discovered the 'secret sauce' to SUP and a new way to enjoy the water and to fuel my addiction to being salty!

It seemed so easy. And in some ways, it was. Everyone I took paddling loved it, especially the journeying aspect. Even my most die-hard ocean-loving friends admitted there was something special about it. Better still, unlike windsurfing or surfing – where teaching a beginner often meant sacrificing your own session – SUP allowed everyone to enjoy it together, instantly. It was as easy as riding a bike.

But there was a hurdle, the board itself. The fibreglass boards were massive, heavy, fragile and a nightmare to transport and store. At twelve-and-a-half feet long and weighing eighteen kilograms, lifting them on to a car was a workout, and finding space at home was tricky. People loved paddling but hesitated to invest in a board. It was a problem.

Then came another lightbulb moment.

In early 2008, I discovered a small California-based start-up making and selling inflatable SUP boards. They seemed to solve the transport and storage issues while still paddling well. I formed a new plan: import and sell them in the UK and maybe Europe. But when I reached out to the owner of the US brand, he flatly refused. He barely even replied. I hadn't anticipated that. That flat *no* profoundly changed the way I saw my life going. It was an almost instant decision. I was no longer going to sell someone else's product and be constrained by their ambitions or lack thereof. I was, with the help of Dave Hackford and Roger Tushingham from Tushingham Sails, going to embark on the next chapter that was to massively influence my life and the progression of the sport of SUP.

So that was that. We set out to develop our own brand of inflatable SUPs. I forged connections with material producers in South Korea and, within six months, created a product that was just about good enough. By late summer, we had a name – Red Paddle Co – and launched into the market. The global adoption of inflatable SUPs had begun.

The journey was far from smooth. While we had solved the storage and transport problem, a new challenge emerged – people didn't believe inflatable boards could perform well, they were seen as gimmicks. The early years were tough, but we stayed focused. We kept innovating, refining and proving that inflatable boards were not only practical but also performed at the highest level. We redesigned the whole package from the ground up, developed new materials, new ways of doing things.

Meanwhile, SUP had become a real addiction for me. I ran Europe's first-ever SUP competition, developed an indoor racing concept at the London Boat Show – a world first – and raced in locations across the globe. I surfed SUPs in legendary spots like Teahupo'o in Tahiti, Chicama in Peru and all over Europe. Windsurfing faded into the background, without me really noticing. SUP had taken over my life, and building Red Paddle Co became my singular entrepreneurial mission.

From a small start-up to the world's leading premium inflatable SUP brand, the journey has been unforgettable. Today, more than ninety per cent of the SUP market is inflatable; a concept that was once doubted, now dominates. The hurdles never stopped coming, but neither did my belief in the sport and Red Paddle Co.

I still think back to those early days, paddling up the river, realising the potential right in front of me – a route I must have now paddled over a hundred times. That moment of exploration not only shaped my personal journey but helped shape the entire sport. The people I've met along the way, the places I've seen and the lessons I've learned have been priceless. My life could have taken a very different path had I not trusted my gut. SUP was something special – something worth fighting for. And it still is.

DESIGNING FOR INCLUSIVE PADDLEBOARDING

WILL BEHENNA

On my way home I reflected on how far I'd come. From those dark days lying in a hospital bed at sixteen, having been told I would never walk again. Here I was at fifty-two, still 'kicking ass and taking names'.

19 June 1988 was a sunny day in Cornwall. I was sixteen years old and in the middle of my GCSEs. The plan for the day was a long cycle ride as part of my training for the Fowey Triathlon scheduled for later that summer. Little did I know that three hours later my whole life would be shattered into a thousand tiny pieces, and I would be travelling down a road far less travelled.

I don't remember anything about the accident although I was conscious. I am eternally grateful to the ambulance crew who arrived shortly after I cycled into the back of a stationary car. They instantly realised how seriously injured I was and refused to move me until the air ambulance arrived and flew me to Derriford Hospital.

I had crushed my spine, split my sternum (supposedly the hardest bone in the body to damage) and had major lacerations all over my head. There were fears of a major brain injury (cycling helmets were not a thing back then), that I had punctured my heart and that I had broken my neck. I remember people coming to visit me in hospital, but everything was incredibly fuzzy. A week later I was driven by ambulance to the spinal unit in Cardiff. I lay in bed for ten weeks with little idea what was really happening, how my life had fundamentally changed. Six months later I left hospital in a wheelchair, paralysed from the chest down – no feeling and no movement. I had to relearn how to manage a body that was now completely alien to me. My parents and sister, along with my extended family and friends, were there with me every step of the way but this was *my* journey and at the age of sixteen I had little idea of what lay ahead.

Fast-forward thirty-five years and I'm lifting my paddleboarding kit out of the back of my car ready to go paddling independently for the first time in my life.

Experiencing a spinal cord injury takes you on an incredibly powerful journey. It tests the very fabric of your being. Your body becomes a disaster waiting to happen – you have to learn how to manage your bowels and bladder and understand how to look after your skin which is vulnerable to pressure sores. You experience spasms that can throw you out of your wheelchair and pain in the parts of the body you can still feel. In my case from my chest upwards.

And this is before you start dealing with the psychological impact. Realising you're never going to walk again or play football or rugby with your mates. The phrase 'you don't know what you've got until its gone' rings in your ears. Back then there was no mental health support, no counselling on offer, and talking about what had happened just felt so intense. Even now I look back and have no idea how I got through those dark years. But nine months after my accident I was driving a car, playing table tennis for a local club, swimming at the local pool, planning to go back to college to do my A-levels and randomly was helping shape windsurfing boards down at the local beach.

I had always been drawn to the water. I grew up on the beach and being out on or in the sea always felt special. So, within twelve months I was on the water in a kayak. It was a real challenge to get on the water; there were no facilities, and I was wobbly as hell, but I reconnected with the water. It would be another two years before I went kayaking and sailing with an amazing spinal injuries charity called The Back-Up Trust. They provide outdoor adventure courses for people with spinal injuries, and I just loved it. That was the springboard for the start of my kayaking adventures.

Disability paddling was still in its infancy, but I connected with some amazing people and over the years became a competent paddler, learning how to carve foam to make seating systems so I could improve my paddling ability. I also loved helping other people with disabilities get out on the water. However, due to my injury, it was impossible for me to roll a kayak, and I could never pick one up to put it on the car, making it impossible to get out on the water on my own. I was always reliant on other people.

A major part of recovering from spinal injury is re-establishing your independence. Everything for me centred on being independent. So even though I loved being on the water, whether it was sailing, waterskiing, scuba-diving or kayaking, I craved being able to do it solo.

Fast-forward to 2021 and we were all experiencing lockdown and desperately trying to find activities we were allowed to do. I don't even know how I came across paddleboarding but there it was, this wide, flat and stable floating platform, and more importantly it was portable. I looked at it and thought, 'You know what, that might work.' My paddleboarding journey had begun.

I started looking at seating options but soon realised that nothing was going to work for me. Fabric seats provided no postural or lateral support, so I went out and bought a paddleboard and set about building a seat. The first prototype, made of plywood, was tested down in Cornwall three months later, and it worked. The next version, made from closed-cell foam, was a significant improvement and made me realise independent paddling was possible.

What I found so empowering about paddleboarding was the community. I'd experienced negativity and disinterest from several kayaking clubs over the years. The paddleboarding community was the complete opposite. They were so welcoming and accommodating. I couldn't quite believe it and soon realised I had found my tribe.

So, in June 2023, having spent countless hours on the water, growing in confidence and constantly evaluating the feasibility of paddling independently, I hatched a plan. Fortunately, four miles from my house I found the perfect launch spot on the River Stour. I'd paddled there many times so knew it would be well within my paddling capabilities. So, one afternoon I rocked up and grabbed my kit out of the car. I then connected all my gear and fixed a set of kayaking wheels on to the back of the paddleboard. I then lifted the front of the paddleboard on to my lap and secured it around my waist using a climbing sling. Then I carefully manoeuvred my paddleboard, on the wheels, down to the water's edge before transferring from my wheelchair on to my paddleboarding seat. I had made a poster which I pinned to my wheelchair stating: *I am an experienced paddleboarder, please do not move my wheelchair, I will be back in an hour. Enjoy your day.*

As I paddled upstream, initially it felt just like another paddling trip. However, paddling through a reed bed, I stopped and absorbed my surroundings. The silent flow of water; the trees dancing in the wind; the clouds gliding overhead. Then it dawned on me. I had waited a lifetime for this moment and here I was making it happen. I posted on Instagram and then continued my adventure, a sense of tranquillity washing over me.

On my way home I reflected on how far I'd come. From those dark days lying in a hospital bed at sixteen, having been told I would never walk again. Here I was at fifty-two, still 'kicking ass and taking names'.

Six months later I set up Inclusive Paddleboarding with the specific intention of supporting people with a range of different medical conditions and disabilities (i.e. those who have difficulty standing) to get out on the water. I want everyone to experience the connection with green and blue spaces which, to this day, still has such a profound effect on me. I have refined and developed my designs, creating a kneeling seat, beach matting and a paddling system for people with limited arm function.

I can see so much potential. I have plans in place to:

- Establish eight Inclusive Paddleboarding venues across the country.
- Start a campaign to improve beach access for people who are currently excluded from the beach environment.
- Develop a paddleboarding active rehab programme for people who have experienced a traumatic injury.
- Qualify as a paddleboarding instructor.
- Complete a week's paddleboarding adventure in the Norwegian fjords.

I know how important being on the water is for my physical and emotional well-being. A place of calm, the opportunity to see the world from a different perspective, that feeling of freedom and independence and the perfect opportunity to connect with like-minded people. Paddleboarding has given me so much in such a short time. Working with so many amazing people across the UK and Europe I will continue to find innovative solutions that can enable and empower everyone to feel what I feel when I'm on the water. Please reach out if you have any ideas or want to get involved.

MAKING A DIFFERENCE
ADYA MISRA

I have realised when I wake up feeling exhausted after a bad sleep or perhaps a long week at work, my energy and vigour returns as soon as I'm on the water. For me, it's magic.

'You're going paddling again?' my mum used to ask me when I would mention going kayaking over a weekend when she had made plans for us together. At that time, I was in Dorset every other weekend for sea kayaking, after multiple kayaking or canoeing trips on the River Thames with new friends. In hindsight, I can see why she asked.

When I started kayaking in Lake Mälaren in Stockholm it was a weekday activity that no one questioned. It was the Swedish summer staple, and I suppose everyone assumed I was going native. Weekly organised trips turned into multiple trips during the week, and no one questioned it. 'It's great exercise,' everyone told me. I never showed any interest in sport when I was a child, and my parents never pushed me to sport either. Family and friends were surprised, but supportive of my new hobby. 'Your photos always look amazing,' they would say. The light in the summer evenings was spectacular, and the setting sun turned the lake orange. As the waves tested my balance, I was mesmerised by the beautiful sights and smells of the city from the water.

There was a shift when I returned to the UK and joined a kayak club. There were regular weekday paddles, multiple weekends away and everyone in my life stood up and noticed. While I was learning everything about paddling, tidal planning, assessments and camping, I simply didn't have the same interest in or time for leisurely walks, window shopping or coffee dates. Since I was new to the sport, all my conversations were centred around my favourite places: the River Thames and the South Coast.

People often talk about the health benefits of taking up a sport or making outdoor pursuits a bigger part of your life to encourage more folk to get outdoors. We've all heard and seen news stories and research articles that percolate down to Instagram stories, TikTok videos and influencer diaries. All of the research and personal stories are true – the outdoors will change your life.

After all these years I have realised when I wake up feeling exhausted after a bad sleep or perhaps a long week at work, my energy and vigour returns as soon as I'm on the water. For me, it's magic. Feeling the lilt of the waves and watching their patterns dancing around me keeps me grounded. Bigger waves are more humbling, and windy days are a test of my mental resolve. The smiles are sometimes a bit tired but always very big.

The stories that remain untold are the ones of loneliness, and confronting the truth about changing your life when you start something new and the sense of loss when the people in your life don't join you in your new pursuit. Add to that the realisation that you're the only person of colour in the group. What is the collateral damage?

Since none of my friends or my family paddle, I've had to find new friends and make new connections, while nurturing relationships with people who loved me when I didn't have paddle sports in my life. I often have to make tough choices on how to spend a beautiful day – between spending time with my loved ones and paddling. I started the grassroots movement People of Colour Paddle in 2022 to encourage more people to try paddle sports. I run kayaking and paddleboarding sessions in small groups to get more people involved and help them to step outside their comfort zone. When running these sessions, it became clear to me that I had changed so much since I started paddling.

In every person attending sessions with me, I saw a version of me before I started paddling. Some were really excited until they had to get their feet wet, others embarrassed to do something silly or simply too scared to be near water. Many people didn't want their photos online because they felt their families wouldn't understand.

But, once everyone's worst fears didn't come true and we ended up sharing a lovely couple of hours on the water, there were smiles all round.

Unlike many others who discovered the joy of being outdoors over the pandemic years, those years helped me and my family to fully understand why there were quite so many paddling trips. When things were uncertain, or in flux, paddling was my constant. My anchor. That's when I properly got into paddleboarding too; kayaking was trickier at that time because I didn't have my own boats and couldn't access the boats at my club as much due to the restrictions in place.

I had my first group lesson in September 2019 with Liverpool SUP Company. After messing about on my own during lockdown, in April 2021 I had some excellent coaching and consolidated my skills in paddleboarding on flat water. The paddleboarding community was getting bigger at that time – everyone seemed to have a board! I was completely hooked on paddleboarding and I remember running three or four sessions a week for my canoe club. I've got no idea how I managed that now, but it helped me qualify as a paddleboarding coach a year later in 2022.

Now, my mum gets it. When I tell her I'm going for a paddle, she just says, 'Have a great time, and send photos.'

HEALING: MY CANCER JOURNEY

MELODY SMITH

Paddleboarding didn't just help me heal – it gave me back my life. It introduced me to a world of adventure, an appreciation for living in the moment and the unparalleled healing magic of blue and green therapy.

The sky stretches out above and beyond, a blanket of dull blue-grey blending seamlessly into the slate-blue sea. At first glance, it seems cold and uninviting – a scene better suited for storms than this perfect serenity. Yet here I stand, a wave of triumph washing over me. The air is warm, embracing me, as the first gentle drops of rain fall, forming tiny ripple kisses on the glass-like surface of the sea. I feel more alone than I ever have, yet more at peace and content than I have ever hoped or wished for. Alone with my thoughts, I stand – triumphant, in awe that I am balancing on a paddleboard, floating between sky and sea.

Eighteen months ago, I stood in a consultation room in hospital, searching my doctor's face for a clue as to what she was about to tell me. She invited me to sit on the single chair pulled up alongside her desk, while a Macmillan nurse hurriedly pulled up a second chair next to it for my partner. Up until this point I had been quietly confident that it would be welcome news — after all, the chances of this strange little lump in my right breast being cancer seemed so slim. Twenty minutes later I left that office numb in the knowledge that I was the one in two, a statistic.

I approached my battle with cancer head-on, armed with my artillery of positivity. I knew I needed to be strong – not just for myself, but for my family. Through the months and months of chemotherapy, surgery and radiotherapy, I held on to hope and the belief in a positive attitude breeding an army of positive cells within me, within my body and mind. Finally, the moment came for me to ring the bell, the bell that is mounted on a wall at every cancer treatment unit, like a beacon of hope and a symbol of life, the ultimate goal. I had heard it toll several times during the course of my treatment. Each time my heart swelled in relief and pride for the survivor signalling they'd won their battle, and for eight months I wanted nothing more for myself and my family than to ring that bell at the end of my cancer journey. Finally, I rang that bell crying tears of joy. A week later confirmation in writing arrived: 'No evidence of disease.' I had imagined I would feel relief, elation or pride.

I felt helpless and afraid. In fact, terrified.

From diagnosis up until that point, I had been monitored, tested and scanned regularly. Every little change happening inside my body was tracked and treated. Then I rang that bell, said all my thank yous, hugged all my NHS angels, walked out of those doors and realised I was now on my own with this invisible threat. My body would now only be monitored by me – no blood tests or scans. My senses and intuition would be scanning for any little change that could potentially mean the return of this aggressive type of cancer. The fear of not knowing if it had returned terrified me more than the initial diagnosis itself.

The irony and cruelty of feeling more afraid after beating cancer than I did when I had it, destroyed my inner strength and positivity. My positivity was sadly becoming more and more of a facade. I knew I needed to find something to pull me forward and keep me from dwelling on the what ifs. I love the sea and always dreamed of taking up a water sport. My appalling sense of balance ruled out surfing and the speed of windsurfing or kitesurfing felt too daunting. It was during the first Covid lockdown that an unexpected opportunity presented itself and rescued me.

My son-in-law had bought my daughter an inflatable stand-up paddleboard, and during the summer of 2020, he made it his mission to find the quietest beaches on the South Coast where our family bubble could escape to the seaside once the Covid restrictions allowed us to.

On 16 August 2020 it was remarkably quiet on West Wittering Beach. The sea was calm, my mind was not. I can recall the frustration of realising I should be relaxed and happy to be with my family on a lovely beach, watching the sea and celebrating the fact that I was almost a year on from my chemotherapy and surgery and in remission. As I lay on my beach towel, gazing out at the sea, my eyes fell on the paddleboard resting in the sand just beyond the sandcastle my grandchildren had built. I had thought about trying it before but always talked myself out of it. This time, before doubt could creep in, I stood up, walked over, and asked my daughter and son-in-law if they minded me giving it a go.

As I paddled out, I lost track of time. Sitting on the board, staring into the horizon and soaking in the tranquillity – the rare peace of a mind unburdened by fear or anxiety. At first, I had no intention of making a fool of myself by attempting to stand. But curiosity got the better of me. I tried several times, each attempt ending with an ungraceful splash into the water. The sea was calm and warm enough to be inviting but cool enough to be refreshing. I was enjoying the dips and the challenge each time to climb back on the board.

Then it happened, I stood up and I stayed up. My legs trembled; my body was so tense I thought my legs and back might seize into a cramp. I dipped the paddle into the water, and the board and I moved forward. I was still standing. I was stand-up paddleboarding! As I picked up some speed my legs stopped shaking, my breathing calmed and my body relaxed a little. As I looked out into the vastness of the slate-blue sea, the raindrops began to fall, gentle and rhythmic, as if nature itself was celebrating with me. That was my moment – the moment I found the new me.

From that day on, I was hooked. My mother, sensing the positive impact it had on me, gifted me my own paddleboard for my birthday. It became my escape, my therapy, my joy. My new passion and my new life.

I was by no means a natural, but that was part of the beauty. Paddleboarding welcomes all levels, and even the most experienced paddlers take unexpected dunks. I soon discovered the warmth of the SUP community – no judgment, just encouragement, laughter and adventure. I joined a local group and embarked on expeditions on the River Wey, the Basingstoke Canal and the River Thames.

My first social paddle turned into an eight-hour endurance challenge to a pub and back. The wind had picked up and changed direction, making our return journey an unexpected challenge, every one of the six of us having to dig deep to make it back to the launch spot before dark. We struggled, we laughed, we may even have cried, but we made it back together.

We all learned lessons that day and I learned that my mind was no longer overwhelmed with dark thoughts of my cancer returning and the fear of not knowing until it was too late. I learned that I was able to live and breathe with a positive attitude once again. I fell in love with SUP which in turn enabled me to refocus and fall in love with life again.

What could have been the darkest years of my life have been the lightest and brightest years filled with discovery, adventure, friendship, unexpected physical and mental skills and strengths, and an overwhelming joy for life. I had just ended a toxic relationship, completed a gruelling year of cancer treatment, moved house and was shielding because I was considered to be a highly vulnerable person. Yet, through it all, I found solace on the water.

Ask anyone who takes to the water, and they'll tell you, the moment you're floating and your paddle dips into the water, a switch flips. Worries dissolve, stress fades and all that remains is the rhythm of the paddle and the water and the feeling of being embraced into nature.

Paddleboarding became my antidote to post-treatment anxieties, my fuel for positivity. Through it, I have made incredible friendships, found confidence and embraced life with a renewed sense of adventure and confidence.

In 2021, inspired by the NHS that saved my life, I embarked on a new career in the ambulance service. I have introduced SUP to my colleagues, and now I have a fantastic group of paddleboarding buddies at work who enjoy the same mental health and well-being benefits that I do.

My love for stand-up paddleboarding is fuelled by its incredible versatility and variety. Many of our paddles include a well-earned halfway pub stop (because, why not?), but whether I'm paddling for exercise, solitude or social connection, every outing feels like a gift. Some days, I simply lie back on my board, drifting gently as I take in the world around me – watching birds flit through the trees, admiring the water's magical reflections, rescuing struggling bees and marvelling at the fearless damselflies that land for a rest.

Other times, I paddle with purpose, pushing my body to feel the full benefits of an activity that engages every muscle, or I challenge myself to master a new skill or technique. Even on social paddles, there's always the freedom to forge ahead or hang back – finding space for quiet reflection and wonder.

Paddleboarding didn't just help me heal – it gave me back my life. It introduced me to a world of adventure, an appreciation for living in the moment and the unparalleled healing magic of blue and green therapy. Now, as I step into another adventure of a new and promising relationship, it fills me with joy to know he is keen to buy a board and start planning SUP adventures with me for the future.

I know SUP will always be a part of my life. SUP helped me build resilience, rediscover joy and embrace the beauty of the present moment. Cancer changed me, the NHS saved me and SUP set me free. As long as I have my board and my health, I know I'll always find my way forward – one paddle stroke at a time.

BLUE HEALTH AND BLUE SPACES

CLARE OSBORN

Focusing on glimmers instead of worries acts almost in the same way as a gratitude practice might. This is a useful tool to help us to shift our state of mind, just as the ocean shifts from wild waves to calm seas.

'She might not make it through the night.' I was struggling to absorb the words ...

My mum had been blue-lighted to A&E two days before and was now in ICU in an induced coma. It felt like a nightmare. My world had been turned on its head and nothing has been the same since.

Mum ended up spending two months on life support fighting for her life. Two months of not knowing if she would live or die was devastating. Survival mode kicked in and I found myself reaching out for help, something I didn't really do. A friend offered me a paddleboard at cost price and suggested that I make sure I took time out for myself.

Getting on a paddleboard felt like a stretch but I started a routine of getting myself to the beach every day. At first just to watch the water, which seemed to make this hugely traumatic experience feel somehow manageable. Watching the waves seemed to melt the stress out of my body. I knew at that moment that I needed to spend more time in these blue spaces and resolved to get out on that shiny new SUP as soon as I could.

Through paddle sports I found solace in the water, watching the ripples of my paddle and the drip-drop of water as it broke the surface.

I got lost in the reflections of the clouds in the river and the ever-changing textures and colours of the riverbanks. Watching the seasons flow as baby ducks got ferried along by their mums, picking the blackberries in summer and braving the cold frosty banks in winter.

I later learned that noticing all these 'glimmers' helps us to regulate our nervous system, and it is a scientifically proven way of reducing stress and increasing well-being. Focusing on glimmers instead of worries acts almost in the same way as a gratitude practice might. This is a useful tool to help us to shift our state of mind, just as the ocean shifts from wild waves to calm seas.

After living through that traumatic experience with Mum, going back to sit at my desk in my corporate job as a real estate lawyer felt a bit meaningless. I'd been fighting low-level depression for years, trying to mould myself into corporate life and numb myself from this 'nature-disconnected' way of being. I realised I would burn out if I stayed and without a plan I jumped into the unknown.

An opportunity arose to do some epic conservation paddle expeditions and so in three consecutive years I ended up paddling the width of Britain, length of Wales and in remote Scottish Isles to clean plastic out of these spaces and raise awareness about plastic pollution.

I started to experience the devastating impact humankind is having on these spaces that are so vital for our mental health. I remember sitting on a beach in the Summer Isles and seeing rare birds' nests filled with blue and green strands of plastic fishing nets and crying.

The pandemic couldn't have come at a worse time. It not only had a devastating impact on my mental health, but I was in the process of launching a business as a blue health and mindfulness coach. The bizarre and unprecedented lockdowns we were thrown into left me struggling to hold counsel for myself, let alone hold space for others online.

I also felt guilty because I wasn't being a perfect eco-human. I felt overwhelmed by the issues we were facing, and grief for the natural world that we are losing before our very eyes. I felt conflicted between wanting to talk about ocean plastics and sustainability, but also immensely aware of the need for all to connect and to heal. It all started to come together when a coaching client of mine suggested I became a SUP instructor. So that's exactly what I did!

I now regularly run lessons and river trips and have found a way to weave conversations about our interconnectedness with nature into these experiences. Getting my group anchored in a circle lying on their backs on their boards and guiding a meditation, watching the stress roll off their shoulders and into the water, into Mother Earth, where she can hold what feels like too much … is truly humbling. I noticed early on how people find it easier to open up and be vulnerable in these spaces. The water gives us permission to spill our thoughts and feelings out into it.

It's not just stress that I see left behind in the water, it is self-doubt too. People arrive for their river adventure convinced that they're going to spend the day on their knees or fall in. Not that there's anything wrong with doing either of those things. All bodies are different and if you need to spend the day sat on your bum and using the paddle as if you are in a canoe, so be it – you do you! But what is amazing is to see that self-doubt turn into self-power, as it did for me. And I love to then ask: 'If you didn't think you would be able to do this, but have, what else are you not doing because you "think" you can't?'

I always believed I wasn't sporty but now I teach a water sport – who would have thought that, definitely not me! And if I can do it, I know you can too if that's what you want to do. But to me it's more than a sport, it's a vehicle to get out into nature, into blue spaces. To pause and be present. And if in that day of adventure and paddling and trying something new, you also start to understand that you are part of this ecosystem that you are floating along in, and not apart from it, that the atoms we breathe are the same as those that make up the water that we float on and the myriad of colours and textures around us, then I feel like I am doing a little bit of good in the world.

Being out in nature wasn't the only thing that helped me to recover, having a purpose and a passion did too. Volunteering introduced me to a community and helped me to feel like I was part of something bigger than me. I'm now fortunate to be employed by the UK charity Surfers Against Sewage, getting to support incredible volunteers to do amazing things to protect our waterways. Volunteering has literally changed my life and my career path, and I feel honoured to work in this sector. It's not been an easy journey mind you, there have been many bumps along the way. I had to move into my van as the drop in income meant I couldn't afford to live in the south of England any more. But I now see all these things as a sign that I'm supposed to take a different path and live in a different location in the UK. Wilder places are calling me so watch this space!

I've also realised that the guilt around not being a perfect eco-human is super common – I regularly hear it from the volunteers I work with. I've now let go of this unachievable goal. I advocate 'progress over perfection' and just doing what's right and what works for you. So, let's try not to judge ourselves and just do what we can while getting into nature or on to the water as much as possible and supporting others to do the same. The more we connect to our wild spaces the more we come to understand them. And to quote Uncle Ben from Spiderman: 'With great power comes great responsibility.' But, of course, with great responsibility comes great power. If we all take a little bit more responsibility for the places we paddle in and the nature spaces we love then imagine the future we might have.

I am eternally grateful to the water for the lessons it has taught me and the teachers that have encouraged me to do things beyond my comprehension. What started as a need to get out into nature to heal from trauma gave me a whole new perspective on what I could or couldn't achieve and ultimately became a new career for me. And as for Mum, well it's now ten years on and she gets out into nature on walks as often as she can. She's even sat on a paddleboard in her seventies – and after an experience that left her having to learn how to eat, drink and walk again. During lockdown she did couch to 5K, and has just relocated home to the Isle of Man. So, I now get to explore the wild coasts of her new home and continue to feel awe inspired by the strength of my beautiful mum.

PADDLEBOARDING PODCAST

SIMON HUTCHINSON

For me, paddleboarding has been a profound life experience. It's soothed and provided therapy, helping me to keep going through some long and very tough periods in my life, and these sessions with Sean have been central. Off the water, it's grown into a creative opportunity for me to share my love of this sport with others, through my podcast.

It's early morning. I'm sitting in my car with my board still on the roof, as I wait for my friend Sean to join me.

I'm parked in Keyhaven, an ancient Hampshire fishing village at the mouth of the Solent where, to my delight, I've bagged one of the four highly prized parking spots directly by the quay. In front of me is the slipway where we've launched so many times, and looking to my right across the salt marsh I can see Hurst Castle and the top of the Needles Lighthouse behind the protective shingle bulk of Hurst Spit.

Being a member of the paddleboarding tribe is a privilege which has given me so many incredible memories and experiences, but there is something very special about this place.

As a gentle orange glow appears across the horizon in front of me, Sean, my longstanding paddle partner and someone I've shared so many experiences with on the water, triumphantly pulls his car into the final parking space right next to me.

We've been getting out on the water together for over ten years. Both of our lives have changed dramatically since we first met back in 2014, but paddleboarding has remained our shared passion and has given us plenty of memorable experiences.

Many of them started from this exact launch point and on this water. This was the place where I first started going out on to the water, solo and inexperienced. It was the place where, many years later, we set out on a down-winding adventure in gusts of over sixty miles per hour to a destination we reached in twenty minutes, rather than the traditional ninety for a less wind-assisted journey.

This was also the place where I qualified as an instructor, where races were held, where there were demonstration events and skill sessions, and where we went out to do exactly what we were doing today, just getting out and experiencing the beauty of the water.

For me, paddleboarding has been a profound life experience. It's soothed and provided therapy, helping me to keep going through some long and very tough periods in my life, and these sessions with Sean have been central. Off the water, it's grown into a creative opportunity for me to share my love of this sport with others, through my podcast.

As we carry our boards to the slipway, the sun has partially crept out from behind the Isle of Wight, flooding the quay with low but bright and powerful light – I can feel its warmth on my face as we pause and take it in. We both know that these moments don't last long, and I try to freeze it into my mind by drinking in the detail, noticing the clear glassy water, the sounds of the seabirds and the family of swans swimming hopefully towards us.

The famous 'philosopher' Ferris Bueller once said, 'Life moves pretty fast. If you don't stop and look around once in a while, you could miss it', and it's very clear to me that the joy of paddleboarding is tied up into exactly these moments.

It's not just my own experiences which tell me that – it's a common thread which runs through all the conversations I've had with guests on my podcast. Regardless of the level of extreme athletic, endurance or personal objectives they've overcome, it's never simply 'achieving' which emerges as the most important factor – it's about the moments on the water, and the connections made with others and with nature.

This was demonstrated perfectly by podcast guests Barbara and Günter, who paddleboarded 2,000 miles down the Yukon River, through one of the most isolated and wild areas in the world. As well as being awed by the scenery and wildlife, they described their most profound experience of this epic adventure as being the bonding and relationships they formed with the First Nations peoples they met, who showed them incredible hospitality and generosity on their journey.

The objective which you might *think* is the objective, is never *really* the true objective.

Being in, on or near the water is a fundamental basic human drive. In his best-selling book *Blue Mind*, Wallace J. Nichols argued that the premium price of waterfront properties or the soothing mental effects we experience from the sounds and sight of water aren't an accident. Our close relationship with water is hardwired into us as human beings. It's therefore no coincidence that SUP helped people deal with trauma following the pandemic, when it became an effective therapy for so many.

In this dropping tide, we float our boards and wade out into the cold water, being careful not to drag our fins on the submerged slipway. We step on to our boards as the sunrise gains pace and we pull ourselves forward with our paddles, the noses of our boards cutting foamy lines in the glassy surface.

When I first started paddleboarding, it was still a new sport and whenever I was pumping up my board, curious passers-by stopped me to ask me what I was doing.

Picking up a completely new sport later in life aged forty-two also retaught me some important life lessons that I didn't realise I'd forgotten. Most importantly, it taught me that the indignity of falling into the water repeatedly as my body got used to dealing with the motion of the water, waves and swell, was the price that you had to pay to take part. It taught me the patience to accept that falling in wasn't a sign of failure … it was only feedback.

Neptune demanded an upfront investment of time to connect mind and body with the movement of the sea and it was only after paying the admission price and achieving a certain level of competence that I recognised the false assumptions I had made when I'd started. I remembered seeing the effortlessness of others standing on the water and the frustration I felt from being bucked off the board by the most innocent and gentle-looking swell. Thinking that if something looks easy, then it must be easy, is an expectation which is ripe for disappointment and frustration.

I learned from Sean his mantra of, 'If you're not getting wetter, you're not getting better', and this simple rhyming lesson reflects how often we prematurely label ourselves as 'failing' and that we can lose out from giving something up too soon. Any skill which is worth having involves some type of persistence and struggle.

It's a short trip today; we're heading out into the Solent via Hawker's Lake, aiming to drop back into Keyhaven River near Hurst Castle and then back to the quay, but we'll need to keep a close eye on the tides because this area has powerful forces at play, with much of the water becoming mudflats during its tide cycle. I've been here many times before when the tide is dropping quickly … when you're trying to paddle hard against the water, while *also* having to stand up near the nose of the board to raise the fin at the tail, because the water is too shallow to take it.

As we emerge from Hawker's Lake and out into the Solent, we feel the water moving differently under our boards, reflecting where the river meets the sea. We hang a right and continue on until we reach the main channel back into Keyhaven River. We can feel the flow gently pushing against us as we work our way back into the salt marsh. The castle is now in front of us, and we parade past the anglers who've been here overnight in their shelters and are now brewing their tea and being warmed by the morning sun.

It was right here, on a similar idyllic morning, and a 5 a.m. sunrise, when I joined Sean and his SUP team from New Forest Paddle Sports to provide safety cover for a Surfers Against Sewage charity swim to the Isle of Wight. The shortest crossing distance was almost two miles – a serious distance even in the shelter of a pool. But out here, where the water is funnelled tightly between two landmasses as it enters or leaves the Solent, it's a *really* tough swim.

Despite being meticulously planned for the time of year, month and hour when the tidal flow was at its least powerful, from the moment the swimmers set out, they were locked into a growing and disorientating battle to swim at enough of an angle to the flow to avoid being pulled quickly out into the open water of Christchurch Bay, while still making progress towards the island.

I paddled alongside the two swimmers I was assigned to, shouting encouragement as they battled the tidal flow. They eventually reached land, over two miles further along the Isle of Wight coast than the planned landing point.

Being out on the Solent with them at sunrise, witnessing their perseverance and then sharing their jubilation when they made landfall, felt like a real privilege. As we met up with the others – and enjoyed bacon sandwiches and coffee in the morning sun – everyone bonded and connected over this unique shared adventure.

Sean and I turn our backs on Hurst Castle, and we follow the buoys marking the centre of the channel and the route back to our launching point. We've not been out for long, but we can clearly see the water gathering pace as we cross the path of the flow heading strongly from the salt marshes out into the Solent. We lean to the right and raise our rails (sides) to avoid being tipped over.

The end of the morning's paddle is approaching as we re-enter the quay. There will never be another opportunity to do exactly what we've just done. Any water environment has so many moving parts that we'll never see the same sunrise with the same combination of conditions. Everything changes all the time, including ourselves, which is why we should never take today's experience for granted.

That's why Sean and I always finish every paddle by exchanging the same words: 'This has got to be the best paddle we've ever done.' It may not be strictly true, but it is unique, which does make it special … and that is something which should always be celebrated.

FROM CHAMPION ON THE WATER TO STAR BEHIND THE MIC

SARAH THORNELY

Could I have predicted this for myself at the age of sixty-five? Definitely not. Should we all say yes more to potentially scary things? Of course we should.

Sitting in the booth next to one of the biggest media names in the SUP world, mic'd up and ready to commentate on the largest stand-up paddleboarding event in the world, was a proper pinch-me moment and a feeling I will never forget. It was something I guess I had dreamed of for a few years but didn't expect to happen when it did, and it came at the end of a slightly unsettling year for me.

Twelve years previously I had stepped on to a paddleboard and immediately loved it, like many others before and after me. A few months later I needed a lifesaving operation which really focused my mind on getting on with my life once better, and I decided that SUP would be my 'go to' for fun. Fast-forward another few months and after buying my first board, I entered a race and suddenly realised how competitive I was. I stood on that age category podium with a medal around my neck and decided at the age of fifty-two that I would embrace SUP racing.

Over the next five years I entered every race there was, even going over to Paris early on to race on the Seine. This culminated in 2017 when I jointly won the UK SUP National Series fourteen-foot class at the age of fifty-seven. This was not an age category win, but an overall one, and every year that goes by, I become prouder of that win.

Knowing the joy of being part of the SUP community, I wondered how I could stay involved after I stopped racing at the end of 2017. This came in the form of a race director asking me to be part of an events committee, a meet-and-greet friendly face for newcomers to the national series. He was also exploring live feeds and interviews, something that was happening around the world, but not at that time in the UK. I was soon handed a mic and told to get interviewing. Having had no media training whatsoever, I had three things in my favour: people on the SUP race scene knew my face, I was knowledgeable about the sport, and I had no problem chatting to people. Very soon I was asked to take on the live feeds and that is where I felt I came alive – interacting with friends and families who were watching the racing from the comfort of their own homes while I was on a lead boat or pontoon. It was exciting and I loved it.

My husband and I very quickly set up SUPJunkie, a media brand with a cool logo and tag line. I was not sure where we were going with it, but I had a couple of girlfriends telling me to 'make it a thing', so make it a thing we did. I remember standing at our local railway station waiting for a train to take us to London for a huge event; it was going to be a stunningly hot weekend so our new logoed tees would be seen and the rucksack on my back was full of our tech gear. We were officially launching SUPJunkie.

We politely pushed our way into people's noses, grabbing them for a chat on the mic – we managed over thirty interviews that weekend. We talked to some of the biggest names in the sport and they may not have known who we were before, but they did after that. My husband also hustled us on to a boat to cover the tech race in the dock and when the official coverage had technical issues, we carried on with ours.

The whole weekend was such a rush. I had no fear talking to these superstars, paddlers I had looked up to all the time I had been racing, they are just like you and me at the end of the day and love to chat about their passion.

Shortly afterwards, at a qualifying race for the world championships in Poole, my husband casually dropped into the conversation on the way home, 'I think we should go to China'. This is where the world championship event was going to be held in a couple of months time. Again, without overthinking anything, I picked up the phone to the new team manager and suggested we be part of the team – he had seen first-hand our coverage in Poole and immediately agreed.

After a very hectic few months, we spent two weeks in China supporting the team, covering every aspect of their racing and time there, bringing their stories home to friends and family. I am really proud of what we did there. It was crazy busy before too; we helped with fundraising, getting sponsors, video biographies of all the paddlers and *so* much social media. All the team at that time were self-funded including us – that much has not changed in the world of SUP racing.

So, this has been my life pretty much for the last seven years, attending and covering many races in the UK and travelling abroad too including to Poland, France and the USA. I have witnessed the best paddlers in the world doing what they love, and have had the joy of interviewing and writing about them too.

That led on to another new string to my bow. Six years ago, I provided some photographs for *SUP Mag UK*, a very well-known magazine produced in the UK. This was the start of a wonderful relationship and since then I have been writing articles for them. It has led me to meet some great characters, SUP racers, adventurers and even TV celebrity Jordan Wylie who had decided to paddle around the UK for charity. One of my favourites was interviewing Chris Parker of *SUP Racer*, who for ten years was pretty much my hero when it came to covering races live. A legend of the sport, he spoke his mind and had an absolute statistician's mind – it's a piece I am very proud of.

Over the last few years, I have been bumping into Mathieu Astier from *TotalSUP*, who is an incredible and professional media specialist. He covers races all over the world and has been at many world championships. I have – and so has my dear husband – 'nagged' him to get on the mic together. 'For just five minutes,' I would suggest.

Matty and I would often FaceTime and share news or questions, so on one dreary Thursday in November 2024 I picked up his call. He laughed at me for still being in my PJs! I couldn't quite get my head around what he was saying. The International Canoe Federation world championship event that was being held in Florida and starting the following week needed more people on the media team. He was currently the only one. I had definitely not planned to go to this event, but Matty suggested I call them. After I had taken a few deep breaths, I did as I was told. A few messages back and forth between myself and the organisers led to me being offered the chance to go to Florida and actually be paid for it – almost a first!

After my years of talking about SUP racing to anyone who would listen, I would now broadcast to thousands, not only those watching live through the organiser's channel, but we were also being broadcast live on TV in the US with around 100,000 views over the five days of coverage. It's a good job I didn't know that before I went …

From the Thursday call it was a whirlwind of putting my home in order, doing some research on potentially 600 paddlers attending the event and heading off on the Sunday morning to start work that coming week. I wasn't nervous, I was excited, and I was very much looked after by 'Mr TotalSUP' himself and the whole production crew and director. Matty and I did indeed work well together; his knowledge and memory of so many paddlers is exceptional and it was an honour to be on the mic with him.

The year 2024 had brought about a mix of emotions; I had been offered a book deal, which was exciting and fabulous and something I thought I could achieve. Six months later, I realised it was not, and I went back to the publisher to offer them my apology. It was a pretty big 'no', but it felt right.

Another disappointment followed: my self-funded lifestyle could not support an organisation I had been involved in for seven years and they were unable to support me back. My second 'no', and again it felt right.

Sometimes things happen for a reason and dealing with negatives does not always sit comfortably with me. A few times over the last year, I have been blessed with a huge positive coming directly after the negative. I have also since been offered another book deal which is very achievable this time around. Things definitely happen for a reason and the call inviting me to cover that huge event made me value myself and absolutely know my worth. Saying 'yes' is much more fun!

Looking out from that booth, watching the world-class SUP athletes below, and covering the event live on the mic for five full days was a complete high, possibly the best thing I have ever done in my life and a huge reward for all the hard work I have put into a sport that I love with a passion.

Could I have predicted this for myself at the age of sixty-five? Definitely not. Should we all say yes more to potentially scary things? Of course we should. SUP has brought so much into my life – experiences I could never have imagined and many lifelong friends. I certainly cannot imagine my life without it.

UNEARTHING UNITY
GEMMA PALMER-DIGHTON

Yet, amid these trials, laughter echoed across the water, camaraderie blossomed with each shared struggle, and a profound sense of accomplishment took root – two adults finding a sense of play like children.

The air bites, a crisp sting that awakens every sense. A tapestry of frosted grass and diamond-like crystals greeted me on this January day as I stand, paddle in hand, ready to slip on to the icy River Great Ouse. A familiar thought surfaced: this surpasses anything I ever imagined.

Isn't life about discovering unexpected joy, those quiet triumphs that define our success? It's not external validation, but the inner fire, the silent strength found by following your heart. That's my mantra: true success is joy found in the unimaginable, a testament to life's winding paths.

After years of running, cycling and netball, I found an increased passion for the outdoors, fitness and well-being, ignited by an insatiable urge to explore, especially through the simple magic of micro-adventures that could be squeezed into my schedule. That's when I began paddling. This yearning for more – for longer, tougher journeys, for the grit of racing – was the fertile ground where my passion truly began to unfurl. The desire to explore further, faster and for longer drew me into racing and multi-day trips.

Who am I? That's a question in constant evolution. My early career in my twenties presented an opportunity for self-reflection. This period became a catalyst, revealing that my identity extends far beyond my profession and that true confidence emanates from an inner core of strength. Sport became my voice, the arena where I found my might. Having journeyed from runner to paddleboarder, each step along the way – duathlons, cycling, triathlons, hiking – continues to reveal new layers, mirroring the gradual formation of frost crystals, a testament to my growth. In the same way, my identity unfurls and evolves with each stroke of the paddle, step on the trail, push on the pedal and catch of the arm. It's on the water where I think best, often coming up with creative solutions and innovative ideas.

I remember my first paddleboard experience on Grafham Water – wobbly, uncertain, clinging to the paddle like a lifeline, terrified of the inevitable plunge. But then, the exhilarating dunk into the reservoir's clear depths transformed fear into pure elation. The water, once intimidating, became a vast, inviting canvas. Back then, the idea of leading a group, sharing that wonder, seemed impossible. Becoming a Paddle UK #ShePaddles ambassador, and embodying the initiative to increase access to this sport as an agent for change, opened a world of belonging. It ignited my passion to champion diversity, to create space and visibility for global majority paddlers and advocate for greater cultural diversity on the water. Being an ambassador transcended mere visibility and representation of the would-be everyday paddler; it was about recognising potential, discovering my sense of belonging within a community and knowing I could contribute to something larger than myself.

Life's journey, like a meandering river, flows with exhilarating currents and quiet contemplation, constantly testing resilience. On Loch Ness, during a Scottish point-to-point race, a wave of doubt momentarily gripped me, questioning my ability to cross its vast expanse. Although I knew I could finish, I first had to conquer my inner doubts. Even with inner confidence, the challenge reinforced the vital role of mental strength.

As my blade plunges into the icy water, I reflect – paddling isn't just physical, it's exploration, challenge and connection. Each paddle out, a unique journey, offers personal development, mindful presence and brings vigour to my spirit. Like the ever-changing water, I too am in constant motion. I'm drawn to the stark contrasts that define my experiences. From the serene solitude of UK winter paddles on the River Great

Ouse, where frosted willows catch the low orange glow of the sun and my breath hangs in the still, cold air, stands in stark contrast to the utterly unexpected delight of paddling in the US. One of many truly exceptional experiences included sharing a paddle and a picnic with Linda McCoy from CenTex SUP and 2025 president of USA SUP, Austin, floating while watching the Congress Bridge bats emerge at sunset, their cries echoing in the sweltering heat.

Each paddle on the Scottish lochs, especially on Loch Ness, became a transformative lesson, a reminder that even in the face of overwhelming vastness and the changeable UK weather, I am strong and capable. I remind myself that not every paddle is a race; some are about experiencing epic locations and gaining essential skills. On Loch Ness, I came away with improved board skills, mastering the surge of the water, and a deeper understanding of my mental fortitude.

The water has become a mirror, reflecting new dimensions of my identity. It's where I experience the liberating feeling of moving with the flow, the grounding connection to the natural world, the deep satisfaction of learning new techniques and the unwavering support of a nurturing community. The #ShePaddles ambassador programme exemplifies this transformative power, illustrating how community empowers mutual upliftment. It's about creating a sanctuary where women can freely express their strengths and vulnerabilities, and flourish together, supported by allies. When it comes to inspiring paddlers in the community and endurance events, look no further than the steely Emily King (see page 112) and the lightning-fast problem-solver Ben Sykes. You almost have to wonder, with their free-flowing bank of resources, is there anything they can't do or help others to accomplish?

The water is my sanctuary, my place of clarity and purpose, my nirvana! Gliding across its surface, the sun warming my face, the rhythmic paddling – it's pure bliss. And I want to share that feeling, to invite others to experience this authentic connection found on the water. Forget the curated moments, the perfect images; it's about the feel of the water, the birdsong, the connection to something greater than the individual.

Indeed, paddling has gifted me friendships that will last a lifetime, each encounter a testament to the power of shared passion. Take Adrian Warren, for instance. Our paths crossed on a sun-drenched Saturday, during a casual paddle organised by the SUP Huntingdon community I founded. From that moment, we became an inseparable 'SUP family', pushing each other to become better paddlers and accountable for our progress. Many of my most cherished SUP adventures and training breakthroughs have been spent in Adrian's company, from practising in high winds that take your breath away on a reservoir to navigating the scenic River Wye and battling it out on the tidal Paddle Skedaddle course through the Norfolk Broads. He's a great advocate, always reminding me of my capabilities and celebrating my potential. He's also a perpetual 'fast-moving target' – a friendly rival who keeps me striving to close the gap.

Similarly, Stephen Dash, a kindred spirit I encountered by chance on the river, embodied this spirit of camaraderie. As fellow enthusiasts of multi-day paddles, our connection was instant. Our decision to tackle the River Thames, unsupported, on our inflatable SUPs from Cricklade to Teddington, promised a proper adventure. However, nothing could have prepared us for the baptism by fire that awaited. That first day, under a brooding grey sky as fat raindrops pelted down, navigating a labyrinth of narrow streams choked with reeds and fallen trees became our reality. Driven by a shared love of challenge, we hauled our boards over submerged branches, and the unexpected norm of climbing trees and wading became a masterclass in adaptability and resilience, a constant reminder that even the best-laid plans can be upended. Yet, amid these trials, laughter echoed across the water, camaraderie blossomed with each shared struggle, and a profound sense of accomplishment took root – two adults finding a sense of play like children. We learned to rely on each other, to think on our feet and to appreciate the raw, untamed beauty of the river, even in its most demanding moments, the subtle hiss and bubble of the aerated water against the board a constant presence.

Do you know that saying, 'A stranger is just a friend you haven't met yet'? It sums up my experience with the SUP community – the way everyone's open to learning and connecting, and the incredible generosity I've encountered, even outside of my UK travels. Social media became a bridge, linking me to a global community of paddlers. In North Carolina, I had the pleasure of paddling with Roman Kraus and Bryan Worth from Raleigh SUP, exploring a tree-lined lake and catching the wake of speedboats, rising to the occasion and downwinding. Our whoops and hollers echoed across the water as our paddles dipped into its green depths. With speedboats roaring past, I gingerly took on the challenge of riding Bryan's 404 hardboard, a very narrow flatwater board. A big smile spread across my lips as I quickly learned how to balance and brace on what felt like a plank in the chaos. The sheer fun of it made me wish I could have joined them to surf at the coast that weekend, but a flight back to the UK called.

Then there's April Zilg (@aprilzilg). A rare SUP athlete who, despite fierce competition, held all three world championship titles – ISA (International Surfing Association), ICF (International Canoe Federation) and APP (Association of Paddlesurf Professionals) – in 2022. Thanks to Roman and Bryan's encouragement, I connected with her, and she graciously welcomed me to her lake house. Paddling her ISA championship-winning 404 board, I felt a surge of awe. I leaned down, the cool, smooth surface of the deck beneath my fingertips, and traced the stencilled outline of her surname, Zilg, and the bold stripes of the US flag. The board's responsiveness underfoot was reassuring, speaking to its finely tuned capabilities – a piece of kit crafted for a world-class paddler. Her story – starting at twenty-five and achieving world champion status through unwavering resolve – truly resonated, proving that passion, training and dedication can shatter any perceived limitation.

It was a true privilege paddling with Devin Brown (@afrodiskayak), Community Programme Manager at Mississippi Park Connection, and her kayak, *Drip*. A dedicated advocate for Mississippi accessibility, especially within the Black community, Devin and I shared personal stories of race and nature as we navigated the river's shallows, jumping eddies towards the twin city skyscrapers gently rising in the distance. As the sun danced on the rippling surface of the flowing river, Devin pointed skyward: 'Look there, a bald eagle!' As it soared above us, we shared a moment of awe and wonder. In that moment, Devin's rarity became clear to me – her extraordinary drive and ambition making her a formidable force in paddle sports. She shared her inspiring goal: to become the first Black woman to paddle the entire Mississippi, from source to sea, a vision that resonated deeply because of its slave trade history.

Each trip, whether in the US or UK, has been profoundly transformative, enriching my life and sharpening my skills, empowering me to chase podium spots at regional and GBSUP events. Daring to venture beyond my comfort zone and connect with the SUP community has unveiled a world of phenomenal and unexpected paddling adventures.

So, as I step on to the board, the frost of the riverbank crunches beneath my feet. The sun promises warmth, and I push off, ready for adventure. The rhythm of the paddle, the sway of the board, the twinkling frost, the stillness of the water, the warmth of my breath – it's a moment of perfect harmony gliding with the flow. The potency and vitality come from being surrounded by nature.

My story continues to unfold, each paddle stroke writing a new chapter on the water, my personal canvas of triumph. I am a mindful paddler, a natural leader, a cherished friend within our vibrant community, and an integral part of its spirit. Though the ephemeral frost may vanish, the feeling of freedom and connection it sparked will linger, a constant reminder of my unfolding journey and the exquisite beauty of the unexpected. The water remains my sanctuary, and I, its grateful artist, paint my life with the vibrant hues of joy, resilience, and the enduring bonds of belonging.

KNOWING WHERE I AM MEANT TO BE

EMILY KING

To anyone out there struggling, feeling lost, feeling like they'll never find themselves again – I want you to know that you are not alone. There is a way through. And sometimes, that way starts with just one step – or one paddle stroke – towards something new.

I had built what seemed like the perfect life – running a successful horse-drawn carriage business for weddings and living in the beautiful Cotswolds. It was a world of tradition and celebration, and I loved being part of people's happiest moments. But everything changed in July 2008.

THE DAY THAT CHANGED EVERYTHING

It was a sunny summer's day, and the wedding was going smoothly. My horses were well-groomed, the bride and groom were excited to ride on my horse-drawn carriage to the wedding breakfast to receive their guests, and everything seemed perfect. But then, out of nowhere, two large and aggressive bull terriers appeared. At first, the dogs were just a nuisance, nipping at the horses' legs. But things escalated quickly. One dog lunged for my horse's jugular, the other for its leg. Before I could react, one of my horses collapsed.

Panic took over. Both horses, terrified and still harnessed into the carriage, reared and bolted. Sat alone on my seat, I had no control. They took off at speed and galloped flat out through the car park. Ahead, a hedge loomed – they cleared it. In full flight fearing for their lives their only escape was down a country lane. Nothing could stop them, I was terrified ... nothingness, death was calling.

The horses blindly swerved into a farmyard charging full speed at a five-bar gate, then stopping dead with violent force. I didn't. I was catapulted forward, crashing to the ground with force. The impact knocked the wind out of me, and pain shot through my body as I struggled to breathe. Then I remember nothing.

A farmer rushed in and pulled one of the dogs off me. He locked it away and restrained the other. I was left shaken, bruised and in shock. My horses were badly injured – one needed nearly a hundred stitches. But the real damage wasn't just physical. It was psychological. It was the moment everything I had built crumbled.

LIVING WITH TRAUMA

In the days that followed, I tried to go back to normal, but I wasn't the same. Post-traumatic stress disorder (PTSD) crept in. I lay in bed unable to sleep, my mind replaying the events over and over again. The fear was suffocating. I was constantly on edge, terrified of everything. I withdrew from life, struggling to function. My marriage suffered. My business fell apart. Eventually, I walked out. I left everything behind – taking only my horses and a bicycle. I had no idea who I was any more.

I avoided dogs completely. Just seeing one could send me into a full-blown panic attack. I was stuck in survival mode, unable to move forward. Simple things became overwhelming. I couldn't walk into a shop without scanning every corner for a dog. Crowds felt suffocating. I avoided conversations. I felt like a ghost of my former self.

I tried therapy. At first, it seemed to help. Then the nightmares started. I would wake up drenched in sweat, heart pounding. Every loud noise made me jump. Every shadow made my skin crawl. I was exhausted, drained by my own mind. People around me couldn't understand what I was going through; I couldn't communicate, and I felt completely alone.

The isolation deepened, and I found myself spiralling. I had lost my identity. I had always been strong, independent, in control, but now I was a shadow of myself, barely able to function. The fear was paralysing, and I felt like I would never escape it.

Months turned into years, and I struggled to find meaning. I tried to be me, but nothing seemed to fill the void or help me regain my confidence. I had to find a way to heal and rediscover myself, but I didn't know where to start.

DISCOVERING THE WATER

A friend suggested I try surfing. At first, I was sceptical. How could I possibly trust myself in an environment I didn't control? But standing on the beach, looking out at the waves, I felt something shift. The ocean didn't judge me. It didn't expect me to act a certain way. I waded in. The water was unfamiliar, yet somehow calming. I didn't love it immediately, but I felt different. And that was enough.

I kept going back. Surfing led to stand-up paddleboarding and with it came control. Unlike surfing, where I was at the mercy of the waves, SUP allowed me to dictate my own pace. Each paddle stroke seemed to be pulling my soul back into existence. It gave me something I hadn't had in years – a sense of purpose. I wasn't just existing any more. I was moving forward. And then I met Alan.

FINDING LOVE AND PURPOSE

Alan had his own battles – he had survived heart failure twice. He understood what it meant to feel broken. We connected through the ocean, through shared struggles. Eventually, we built a life together in Swansea, where my passion for SUP grew even stronger.

I started competing, training hard and pushing my limits. The woman who had once been paralysed by fear was now racing at an elite level. I became a GBSUP 12'6" technical and distance champion, taking on white-water rapids and ocean challenges I never thought possible. Every paddle stroke felt like a step further from my past, every finish line another victory over my trauma.

But the journey wasn't easy. There were days when self-doubt crept in, when the fear tried to take hold again. I had to remind myself that healing isn't a straight path. I had setbacks, but I kept pushing forward. I refused to let PTSD define me. I refused to be a prisoner of my past.

THE ULTIMATE TEST

In 2022, I set my sights on something huge – an ultra-SUP triathlon around the Isle of Wight. A hundred-mile paddle, an eighty-mile bike ride and a thirty-mile run. No woman had ever done it without stopping. I would be the first.

It was brutal. Paddling through the night for seventeen hours, exhaustion setting in. The bike ride tested every ounce of strength I had left. The marathon pushed me to my absolute limit. There were moments when I questioned why I was doing it. But with every stroke, every pedal, every step, I reminded myself – I had survived worse. I had been in the darkest place imaginable, and I had clawed my way out. When I crossed the finish line, I knew I had reclaimed my life.

A NEW MISSION

Today, I do more than race. I coach, mentor and advocate for mental health. I help others find healing through the water, just as I did. PTSD still lingers, but it no longer defines me. I've learned to live with it, to use it as fuel rather than fear. New challenges sit on the horizon, there is no such thing as 'I can't' any more, just 'why not, let's give it a go … '

I've seen first-hand how water, movement and SUP heals. I've watched people step on to a paddleboard for the first time, hesitant and nervous, and leave the water transformed. I teach them to trust themselves, to find balance – not just on the board, but in life. I remind them, as I remind myself, that healing isn't linear. Some days are harder than others, but the important thing is to keep moving.

If you had told me back in 2008 that I would come out of this stronger, I wouldn't have believed you. But here I am, standing on my board, looking towards the horizon. I am not just surviving. I am thriving.

LOOKING AHEAD

The next challenge is always around the corner. Whether it's another ultra-endurance event, another long-distance paddle or simply helping someone take their first step towards overcoming fear, I'm ready. Because if I've learned anything, it's that resilience isn't about avoiding hardship, it's about learning how to move through it.

I will always carry my past with me. The trauma, the fear, the battles fought in my own mind. But they don't hold me back any more. They propel me forward. And every time I glide across the water, I know I am exactly where I am meant to be.

So, to anyone out there struggling, feeling lost, feeling like they'll never find themselves again – I want you to know that you are not alone. There is a way through. And sometimes, that way starts with just one step – or one paddle stroke – towards something new.

BLUE SPACE HIGHLAND
LEEANNE MACKAY

That's exactly what paddleboarding does for me, it allows me to find myself again – in moments of uncertainty I feel strangely grounded out on the water. It's my safest space, my 'go to', my solace.

On a glorious spring day, sun shining, temperature rising, water still very cold but refreshing, I decided to paddle east out of Nairn into our gorgeous lagoon and find a calm spot to practise yoga on my paddleboard. What I was really looking for was inspiration for writing this piece. I go to the water in every moment of uncertainty. Combining paddleboarding and yoga provides many wellness benefits; through movement of my body, I find stillness in my mind. The gentle sounds of the water against my paddleboard allow me to fully embrace mindfulness. I had hoped to quieten my racing and excited thoughts to enable me to organise and plan them appropriately.

However, as I arrived at the harbour, I found that conditions were not as expected. There was some awesome-looking surf to be played in, so I adapted. I changed my wetsuit to a thicker one as I knew I'd be going in, and I grabbed my Starboard surf SUP. As soon as I entered the water, I got smashed by the surf. In my excitement I had gone straight in instead of around and I was instantly reminded of my love of that feeling of freedom and aliveness as I was thrown from my board into the crashing waves. At times it's more of an exhilarating thrill than actually catching a wave!

What I got that day was so much more than I expected too. I was privileged to share it with the beautiful dolphins that often frequent Nairn. Stopping me in my tracks, I sat and watched their playful antics and mischievousness. I kept at a distance, giving them their space and freedom. But they were keen to play with me, one swimming beneath my board as I sat watching in awe. In that moment, I felt an incredible connection to nature, to something so much greater than I could ever truly comprehend.

I also felt a connection to myself. That's exactly what paddleboarding does for me, it allows me to find myself again – in moments of uncertainty I feel strangely grounded out on the water. It's my safest space, my 'go to', my solace.

Growing up I felt pretty lost and lacking in purpose. A people-pleaser for sure, I never felt I was good enough, always trying to make others happy. Looking back, I understand now that I had a difficult childhood supporting my dad with his mental health struggles, but at the time that was my normal. After my mum left, we became a team, taking care of each other, and my brother too. As I hit my teenage years, I used alcohol and drugs in an attempt to make sense of my overwhelming feelings. This seemed an impossible task. When I married, becoming a wife and a mum to my two stepsons, Connor and Ronan, I found purpose. While my family was changing, I still hadn't quite found my superpower. I needed them as much as they needed me.

I first tried paddleboarding on a family trip to Auckland, New Zealand, visiting my Aunt Maggie with my then husband Andrew and our daughter Jasmin. We were at our favourite beach in Takapuna soaking up the sunshine and enjoying non-stop fun in and around the water. We had some instruction and then enjoyed gliding over beautiful clear waters and enjoying the views of Rangitoto Island. Wow – what fun SUP was!

On our return I ordered our first paddleboards and made it my mission to paddle as often as possible and discover new paddle spots around Scotland too. I've paddled at many places in Scotland, including Loch Morlich, Loch Insh, up to Golspie and Loch Brora, over to Arisaig. At Loch Maree, I stood on an island on a loch, which itself is on a larger island on a larger loch. I've also paddled at Loch Linnhe, Loch Awe, and even as far south as Southend at the southern tip of Argyll and Bute. I've been fortunate enough to see some incredible landscapes from the water, offering a whole new perspective on life, and inspiring me to do more, see more and share more. From finding a sense of calm on the glassiest of waters to the thrill and adventure of catching waves and being thrown off my board, paddleboarding provides me with a blissful comfort I've never known before.

The way paddleboarding really changed my life goes back to one sunshine-filled summer afternoon picnicking with one of my soon to be most treasured friends, Angela, and our daughters, Jasmin and Amy. Angela is most definitely a gentle soul and also driven, headstrong and very intuitive. She suffers from rheumatoid arthritis and osteoarthritis, causing her debilitating impairment of strength and ability. She has good days and very bad days. She also had a very real fear of the water.

We were at a perfect paddle spot out on the Grantown road, near Nairn. I had two paddleboards with me and the girls were enjoying jumping off them into the inviting water. Angela and I sat chatting, then I said, 'Go on, just have a little shot. Paddle on your knees near the water's edge, I'll be right there beside you.' She complains to this day that I nagged at her to try it. One week later she had bought two paddleboards for her and Amy. Her life was changed forever.

Every opportunity we had we were out paddling, adventuring to different locations. Some of our favourites were Findhorn Bay and Loch Glass, but ultimately Nairn had stolen both of our hearts. We've been visited by the most spectacular basking sharks, with thirty to forty of them coming in quite close to feed. Always maintaining a safe distance, I like to sit on my board and watch their leisurely swimming patterns. The sun glistening off their dorsal fins is something to behold.

Angela has often told me how paddling had changed her life, giving her an escape from life's challenges. I was so happy and proud of her for overcoming her fears. Her confidence was growing and soon she would change my life too. During one of our paddles, she turned to me and said, 'Leeanne, you need to become an instructor, you're so good at explaining, reassuring and encouraging people.' I knew she'd support me with the challenge as she'd been there for me at a time when I had made some huge life changes, including leaving a job at NHS Highland.

My mental health had taken a turn; I'd never experienced anything like it in my life. I couldn't look at myself in the mirror; it was a scary time. I did have some understanding after supporting my dad throughout my childhood when he experienced very real lows and very worrying moments of elation. My experience was work-related: stress and the pressure I put on myself. I made the decision to leave my job, feeling so scared but so liberated at the same time.

With a new job and Angela's help, I started putting plans in place for my own wee SUP school. I had incredible support from friends and Andrew, who helped me with planning and lots of practical setting up.

One thing I have always felt is a need to help, almost 'save', people, which I think comes directly from my childhood. So, it really touched my heart when one day Angela told me that I'd not only changed her life, but I'd saved it. She told me about her darkest moments and then taking a deep breath and imagining wee waves crashing into her, throwing her off her board and feeling alive. She said she hadn't felt alive for a long time, and this was just what she needed. She said this was because I had got her into the sea. I felt immense pride for how I had supported her, and I felt such sadness that she felt so low. This confirmed to me my life's purpose. All I want to do in life is show others that peace and happiness can be found out there in our wonderful calming blue spaces.

It was through this kind of feedback that my confidence grew; I was really finding out who I was as a person and exactly what I had to offer others. Paddleboarding was allowing me space and time to see my superpowers. So, I thought, *I can do this. I can show people another route to wellness. It's water for wellness.*

Fast-forward a year and after one season of delivering lessons, Ali Garrow, a sea kayaking instructor and a retired crisis negotiator with Police Scotland, contacted me after seeing my social media page full of how paddleboarding supports wellness. We soon realised we shared a similar vision of providing free wellness sessions through paddleboarding and kayaking. We decided to set up a charity, apply for funding and also set up a referral system. I'd already done some research and using my previous knowledge from working with the NHS, sorting out the referral system would be straightforward. Setting up the charity was a steep learning curve for both of us. From the start I wanted SUP to be accessible and inclusive for all, with no barriers, especially financial ones. Throughout my childhood there wasn't money for fun water sports activities. I wanted to be able to provide these opportunities for young people, to catch them at those crucial tricky teenage years before turning to unhealthy coping mechanisms like I had.

We worked hard, we made many connections with GPs, Paddle Scotland and other organisations offering green space prescribing, who told us they were excited about this project. Blue space prescribing was happening, and we were leading the way!

Blue Space Highland was born, with a board of incredibly knowledgeable and skilled trustees. During our first season we delivered a number of wellness sessions and collected feedback from our participants. We asked them how they felt before their session. Words like 'stressed', 'nervous', 'emotional', 'sleepless' and 'apprehensive' came up. Following their session, common words included 'pride', 'peace', 'mindfulness', 'calm', 'positive', 'safe' and 'inspired'. Some described how the water was so calming that they were able to focus fully on the environment and their experience right there and then, and not on what had been going through their minds before the session.

This was it! We were fully convinced of the benefits of our charity. We accessed funding through the National Lottery Community Fund and Haventus Ardersier Port Community Benefit Fund administered by Foundation Scotland to enable us to continue on with our mission. It was all very exciting.

As I write, we're entering our second season, and we've launched our calendar of events of even more blue space activities. We have learned along the way that we want to be fully inclusive and meet the needs and preferences of everyone. This year, through our providers, we will be facilitating activities including paddleboarding, kayaking, wild swimming, beach yoga and beach art sessions. We understand that people may love the sea but might not want to actually dip their toes in.

My life has changed in so many ways over the past few years and since finding paddleboarding I have found an inner peace that keeps me so grounded. I will strive to connect more individuals with this calming sense of joy that can only be found in, on or around blue space. As I say to everyone: 'paddleboarding will change your life if you let it.'

QUEEN OF THE CANALS

DAISY BEST

I wasn't in a hurry because I wanted to enjoy every moment. I met some wonderful paddleboarders who transformed my goal to reach the end into precious moments of contemplation, joy, warmth and friendship. Those moments will always stay with me as they enhanced my well-being, confidence and faith in human goodness.

'You are going to paddleboard from one side of the country to the other on your own?' asked my wife, Gaynor, with a slightly concerned look on her face. 'Yes, I really think I can do it,' I replied with feigned confidence. Thoughts of how I was going to manage the logistics and whether it was even physically possible for me to achieve were patiently waiting for my attention.

It was 23 January 2023 and the person who was going to join me on the 162-mile paddle from Liverpool to Goole was no longer available. I had my heart and mind set on it, so, before I could even work out how it would happen, I made the verbal commitment to go by myself and for me, that's a done deal. There was something about being in the last year of my forties and asking myself: 'If not now, when?'

I had my first paddleboarding lesson with my friend, Carolyn, and my father-in-law, Ian, in August 2018. The lesson was a birthday present for Carolyn and as someone who has always loved being in, on or near water, I couldn't let her try it without me! I absolutely loved the new perspective gained from seeing life from the river; the willow trees bending in respect towards the water, the heron gracefully taking flight and the seal that had made its journey from the sea popping up to twitch its nose in a friendly 'hello'. After a further lesson in September 2020, delayed by Covid lockdowns and the busyness of life, I bought my own stand-up paddleboard in 2021.

In 2023, I read that the coast-to-coast from Liverpool to Goole via the canals, that I was due to embark upon in July of that year, was a route for 'experienced paddlers'. I certainly didn't feel like an experienced paddleboarder, and I began to question how I could become experienced. I arranged to meet up with Jo Moseley, the first woman to paddleboard this route, for her advice. When I asked Jo how she coped with the most difficult days of paddling, she smiled and said, 'Just focus on one paddle at a time'. She also gave me lots of encouragement and I left with hope that it was possible for me.

When someone is about to embark upon something that pushes them out of their comfort zone, I think that the biggest challenges are those which are hidden, the psychological battles. Am I good enough? Do I have the 'right' to even think that I can do this? Will I make a fool of myself if I don't achieve it? As a counselling psychologist working with people who present with a range of psychological struggles and often horrific life experiences, I frequently witness how such doubts, when given too much credence, can create significant barriers to new experiences. I concluded that all I could do was try, and that change doesn't happen when we don't take those behavioural and psychological risks.

I had never paddleboarded on a canal until one cold February afternoon in 2023 when I launched, on my own, on to the Bridgewater Canal. I had only ever waded through shallow waters to launch so I didn't have a clue how to access my SUP from a height. As I positioned my right knee on my drifting SUP and my left knee remained on the canal side, I knew that I was going in. Moments later, as I thrashed about in the cold water, trying to climb up the slippery, stone canal side, I reminded myself that it might be easier just to heave myself on to my paddleboard that was eagerly floating behind me. With minimal dignity intact and a small audience of baffled onlookers, I composed myself, did a quick self-rescue on to my SUP and set off over the aqueduct as though this was how I always started every paddle, wondering how on earth I would manage to ever egress from my SUP when my paddle was complete. But I did (mimicking a whale on a sandy shore) and subsequently learned a better technique. All of my mistakes have been really helpful lessons – another paddle towards learning more and something to laugh at myself for.

Of course, I was never really going to paddleboard across the UK on my own. Paddleboarding a linear route requires some planning in terms of logistics. Discussing it with my mum and dad, I suggested that I could join Facebook for the first time in my life and connect with other, random paddlers who I could stay with. 'Stranger danger' triggered my mum to say, 'Why don't we hire a campervan and be your helpers?' That became the plan for the latter ten days of the fourteen-day trip while my good friends Kath and Ellie offered to help me from their home city of Liverpool for the earlier part of the journey. Gaynor was a crucial supporter during my training and throughout every adventure I have embarked upon since. She has never failed to believe in me. I am also incredibly grateful to Kath and Ellie and my mum and dad for all of their patience, food, lifts, emergency SUP pump replacement, clean laundry, laughter, cuddles, massages and encouragement. This team are the foundation from which I was able to achieve what I did. I was never really alone.

Something I hadn't anticipated when planning this trip were the connections that I made with others. I wanted to raise money for the mental health charity Mind, and in doing so raise awareness of the need for us all to talk about our mental health and to recognise the infinite psychological and social benefits that being in, on or near water can bring to our well-being. In order to raise money, I promoted what I was doing on social media and joined Facebook groups such as SUP Yorkshire, led by Mike, who was incredibly supportive on and off the water. I decided to let people know the dates, times and launch points for each day and invited people to join me. I was overwhelmed by the response and the generosity of strangers who were willing to paddle with me for a couple of hours, a whole day or, in some cases, a few days. With every person, there were conversations about mental health, and this extended to people I met who walked alongside the canal. It seemed that my chosen charity encouraged people to open up conversations about their mental health or the mental health of those in their family including experiences of depression, schizophrenia, anxiety, trauma and suicide.

On one of the few days that I was paddling alone, I spoke to a man who was returning to walk alongside the canal for the first time after he had been attacked on a canal side, sustaining injuries that had impacted him physically and left him with post-traumatic stress disorder. He was, understandably, very afraid as his hands shook and he scanned for imminent danger. He said he felt able to talk to me because I was on my paddleboard, a distance away from him. This helped him feel safe and, while not providing therapy, I acknowledged that what he was doing, taking one brave step at a time, was incredibly courageous and valuable. This encounter was one of many privileges for me and a reminder of how facing our fears can bring so much personal growth.

I welcomed anyone to join me whether they were new to paddleboarding or very experienced. It was the summer, and it was warm. I wasn't in a hurry because I wanted to enjoy every moment. I met some wonderful paddleboarders who transformed my goal to reach the end into precious moments of contemplation, joy, warmth and friendship. Those moments will always stay with me as they enhanced my wellbeing, confidence and faith in human goodness. I felt so incredibly supported by the paddleboarders who joined me; some have become friends, including Moz with whom I have shared many adventures such as paddling and wild camping from one side of Scotland to the other on the Caledonian Canal.

I have a track record of making my hobbies purposeful and I think my self-worth is enhanced by training for something that has a tangible reward at the end. I developed a purpose for paddleboarding when I trained for the coast-to-coast and that has now grown into a quest to paddleboard every canal in the UK. As I write this, I have paddled over 650 miles worth of canals since that first dip in 2023 and will continue until I have paddled them all. My friend, Deb, and I have committed to paddle at least one canal together each year as have Moz and I. But I also enjoy the peace of paddling canals on my own where I can decompress from my work and exist for a time in a world that feels uncomplicated. Paddling in conversation with Gaynor, who often walks alongside me on the towpath, is another treat.

City, countryside, beautiful, litter-strewn, picturesque, industrial, friendly, lonely, clean, dirty, sunlit, stormy, still, windy, safe, scary, busy or peaceful; canals are a microcosm of life. I can paddle alone or with a group, for an hour or two weeks, in all weather and seasons. It clears my head, brings me joy and exercises my body. It is an obsession, a passion, a place where I can be at peace, my soul food, my challenger and my comfort. I can't imagine life without paddleboarding now.

SUP WITH A PUP
STEPH BARNICOAT

Finally, the wind dropped, and at dawn I headed to Porthpean Beach to paddle in the bay. Being on the water felt incredible; every stroke felt like empowerment; every movement was bravery. The whole experience felt amazing because I was doing it on my own. I was going at my own pace, progressing on every paddle.

I remember the anxiety on that Sunday morning, feeling sick and cold, fearing the unknown. Arriving at Lostwithiel, nerves and excitement were kicking in. As soon as I got on the water, all that anxiety disappeared. I simply felt excited. It was the summer of 2021, and I was embarking on a SUP adventure to paddle one hundred kilometres along the Cornish coast from the River Fowey to the Helford River, to raise money for the charity Seaful.

It was my first time paddling on that part of the Fowey and it was so beautiful gliding with the tide, the sun sparkling amongst the leaves on the trees. The river widens at St Winnow, and I could see the familiar boats near the village of Golant. I paddled around the corner, passing the beautiful town of Fowey. As I approached the river mouth, I turned right heading west into St Austell Bay. The sea and sky were so blue and the sea so flat that on the horizon it was hard to tell where one ended and the other began. I could see Gribbin Tower, and stopped to take a photo. At Gribbin Head, I aimed onwards towards Polkerris.

Focusing on my paddle, this stretch of coastline is one of my favourites, as there are so many coves to stop for a swim. It is always quiet here, so you get the beaches to yourself. After a short food stop and a quick dip on one of the pebbly coves, I continued to paddle towards Par Beach. The paddle between Par Beach and Carlyon Bay has nothing particularly exciting to look at and there were boats and jet-skis, who seemed to have no understanding of how to behave around more vulnerable water users such as paddlers. At the end of Carlyon Bay, I felt relieved and was able to lose myself in the paddle again and enjoy the clear green water, the rugged cliffs and caves. From Charlestown it was a short paddle to Porthpean, my local paddle spot.

I landed at Porthpean Beach for an ice cream and rest. I think there must have been about a hundred people on boards just in the bay. It couldn't have felt more like summer. The sun was still blazing, so after another sea dip and some chill time, I set off towards Pentewan, which was about eight kilometres away. I passed the sea cave and Silvermine Beach, which was busy with other paddlers. Paddling past Ropehaven to Gerrans Point there can be a bit more movement in the water, so as I edged round, I was relieved to see the conditions were good. Phew, no big waves! As there was a slight swell, I kept my eyes focused on the beauty ahead, and with the smooth motion of my board rising up slightly and back down, it felt very rhythmic. I paddled past Black Head, an incredible sight with large cliffs, and then past my dream house behind a secluded beach. Pentewan started to come into view, and the beach was very busy.

I began to lose my balance and rhythm. I only had a few hundred metres left but I felt wobbly and decided to paddle on my knees. It felt good to be back on the beach. I was so tired but excited for day two after completing thirty-three kilometres of my hundred-kilometre paddle challenge.

Like many others, I have always felt a sense of connection to the sea, or what Wallace J. Nichols describes as 'blue mind' – 'The mildly meditative state of calm, peace, and well-being that people experience when they are near, in, on, or under water.' In his book *Blue Mind*, he suggests that spending time with water can positively impact mental health. Growing up, I thought I was the only person to have this positive connection. No one in my family really said anything special about the ocean and no one talked about mental health or well-being.

A quote from Jacques Cousteau that resonates with me is, 'The sea, once it casts its spell, holds one in its net of wonder forever.'

Whatever its spell it led to my passion for the ocean and marine wildlife and encouraged me to study marine biology. I spent many glorious years working offshore in the great big blue. My role was to look out for marine mammals on offshore projects, and if any were sighted, to carry out mitigation. I would be soaking up the magnificent sight of the ocean every day, seeing nothing but the sea. This provided me with my dose of blue mind.

Wanting to progress my career, I traded the offshore world for a more settled lifestyle in an office. It started to become clear that, as a result of this change, my mental health was slowly going downhill. Although I don't really think of those days any more, I remember driving home from work on the A30 and seeing a horrific crash between two vehicles. I cried, wishing it was me. Almost every night involved a bottle of wine – drinking through my misery – although it wasn't really helping. Those months were a very dark part of my life – a lot of drinking, wishing I could slip away, thinking about ways to go without it looking like suicide.

I cannot remember what the push was, but one day I simply decided to buy a paddleboard. I chose one online and drove to Hatha Paddleboards to pick it up. I remember the feeling – I was on such a high. Afterwards I went climbing with my friend Laura, who is a very good climber – I smashed the route, because I was so pumped.

The next day the board lay inflated in my living room as of course it was too windy to go out! I was waiting for the day with both fear and anticipation. Finally, the wind dropped, and at dawn I headed to Porthpean Beach to paddle in the bay. Being on the water felt incredible; every stroke felt like empowerment; every movement was bravery. The whole experience felt amazing because I was doing it on my own. I was going at my own pace, progressing on every paddle.

Paddleboarding became an addiction to me; at every opportunity I would go out. The darkness in my life was fading away. I stopped having suicidal thoughts and everything felt better.

But then the winter months came, and I noticed my mind was moving back to that darker place. I realised it was because I wasn't getting out on the water. I invested in some winter gear and then nothing stopped me. I was feeling more like my happy, positive self again.

I have now been paddleboarding for eight years, and every day I am so thankful for it. Since I started paddleboarding, it truly has had a positive ripple effect in my life, especially in my career. I have become a SUP instructor, written a SUP guidebook for Cornwall and it has given me the courage to move jobs, and I have recently created a professional development course. I honestly can't imagine any of that progress without my connection to the ocean creating positivity in my life.

Paddleboarding has also helped me gain confidence and ignore the anxiety and fear in other ways, such as hiring a car in California to drive the Pacific Coast and buying a van and heading to Scotland for my first road trip. I believe the Steph before paddleboarding would never have had the confidence to do this – that Steph never really did anything alone.

In 2019, a beautiful soul came into my world, my four-legged friend Percy. I never expected to have such a special bond or look cool with a dog on my SUP, but Percy didn't want to be left behind. So now I share my paddles with my favourite companion. I have watched Percy go from a nervous passenger, not moving an inch on the board, to being very confident and walking around it. I do miss the timid Percy – paddling was much easier then!

One incredible paddle we had was at Porthpean, when a grey seal popped up next to us, head out of the water, eyes fixed on Percy. Percy fixated on the seal – the two were almost nose to nose. It was a beautiful moment; one I will cherish. I love the way Percy gets so excited when we see a seal.

Our favourite days are when we can be on the water all day together with the sea breeze in our faces, especially at Par Beach which is our closest dog-friendly beach, or we head for an adventure day out on the Helford River.

The last couple of years have been very challenging for me. My mum was dying, and she wanted to die in the comfort of her own home. It was hard managing my own life, and I was always busy – working, shopping, making sure she had food and fluids at night. Eventually she did allow us to have carers to help. I also wanted to continue with my voluntary work with the British Divers Marine Life Rescue and the Cornwall Seal Hospital where I have been volunteering for seven years. I love seals and the social aspect working with an amazing team of vets and volunteers from all different walks of life. Along with paddleboarding, volunteering became my therapy during this time. Dating and dinners however had to go.

Some days I would paddle hard, battling against a breeze and paddling the stress away. Other times I would go to a favourite beach at Silvermine, to sit and chill, have a quick sea dip and head back to Mum. In the summer, I simply sat on my board captivated by the glittering sea and blue sky, really soaking up blue mind.

Mum passed away in 2024 and I was soon due go to Scotland for work. Percy and I took some time to explore the North Coast 500 road trip, returning along the west coast, where my heart jumped out of my chest. The lochs simply took my breath away – the water was like a mirror, and I was so excited to paddle. Each paddle was healing.

After feeling great on my trip, when I returned home the wind was too high to paddle and I fell into a pit of depression. Looking back, this was the only stage of grief I felt I really experienced. It was a real eye-opener for me. When people are depressed people often say, 'Go and exercise, it will make you feel better.' Every day I said to myself, 'I will go to the gym,' but every day I felt so tired, my body ached and week after week I didn't make it to the gym. I realised that this must be a common feeling for people with depression, living in a constant whirlpool, not able to get out.

Fortunately, the wind finally dropped, and although my body ached and my mind felt numb, I know the effect paddleboarding has on me, so I dragged myself out. Driving to the River Fowey, getting the board ready and putting my gear on was painful, I simply couldn't be bothered. There was certainly no excitement. Nevertheless, as soon I got on to the board, out on to the water – I was paddling with Percy of course – I was so thankful, I cried! I wasn't out of my depression, but I knew it was a start.

Because paddleboarding has had a positive impact on my mental health and well-being, I felt inspired and motivated to help others. In 2024 I started running mindful SUP sessions for Seaful's Vitamin Sea

Project to connect individuals to the ocean for the mental health benefits and nurture stewardship of our ocean.

I am very thankful that I found the courage to start paddleboarding. I am grateful for how it has provided me with such a sense of well-being and my very special relationship with Percy and the ocean.

SCOTTISH FIVE ISLANDS CHALLENGE

LINN VAN DER ZANDEN

'I did it! This is the moment I dreamed up in my pyjamas at home one night, months ago!' For a while I bask in the feeling of achievement and gratitude for the incredible nature on my doorstep, the beauty of these islands and to myself for taking on this adventure. I dreamed of sleeping under the stars by night, paddling among islands and cleaning beaches which could only easily be reached by water, and I was living it.

I look down and see the seaweed dancing underneath my board. The copper tones from the dulse, my favourite type of seaweed to snack on, mixing beautifully with the yellow bladderwrack. It is curious how much more you notice things when paddling; I suppose it is easy to be more present with nothing but the water in front of you. I feel like a kid again.

My gaze turns to the island in the distance. I look at these islands often from the mainland and for a while now had felt a calling to reach them all by paddleboard. A ridiculous idea surely. I didn't know how, or why exactly, but it was a feeling I couldn't shake.

A few months and some research later, I set upon a unique adventure on my doorstep in the south-west of Scotland. The Five Islands Challenge would cover a range of open ocean crossings, marine protected areas and camps on each island over five days. A solo adventure with purpose to raise funds and awareness for an ocean conservation charity. The route was designed in such a way that I could reach and clean remote beaches which were difficult to access from the road; the islands visited would be Great Cumbrae, Little Cumbrae, the Isle of Bute, the Isle of Arran and Holy Island.*

It was 6 a.m. on a calm July morning and I had already packed up from the night before. I knew the weather was going to change that evening, so I left early and planned to hunker down under a tarp later. The crossing between the next two islands was not long compared to some of the other crossings. However, open crossings can be a bit like a false summit where somewhere in the middle the view doesn't change for a while which leads you to question if you have calculated the tide correctly, and if your board is still moving. The thought doesn't last long, as I notice a plastic bag in the water and paddle over to pick it up with my blade. It is a Tesco bag for life. Suddenly, the most elegant jellyfish, a lion's mane with long tentacles, moves alongside my board, contracting its body effortlessly. I'm pretty sure I talk to them a lot when I paddle solo. The seals, the birds, the jellyfish – they make for good company.

I watch it glide away into the distance and admire the sparkle of the sun on the water, take a breath and think to myself: 'I did it! This is the moment I dreamed up in my pyjamas at home one night, months ago!' For a while I bask in the feeling of achievement and gratitude for the incredible nature on my doorstep, the beauty of these islands and to myself for taking on this adventure. I dreamed of sleeping under the stars by night, paddling among islands and cleaning beaches which could only easily be reached by water, and I was living it.

A sailing boat passes and veers off their course a little to come closer and check on me. 'Are you okay?' the skipper shouts with a kind voice. I reply, 'Yes, thank you, nice day for it. Just heading to that bay. I have my VHF if I need it.' Afterwards, I hope I didn't sound too offended. I like that people check on you; it's such a lovely caring community on the water and it helps make me feel safe. My dad had a little sailing boat when I was young, and he probably would have done the same thing. But I also want to prove to this gentleman that I have a plan A, a plan B and even a plan C if I need it! I already had SUP qualifications for exposed waters and had taken a VHF exam; to specifically prepare for

---

* Little Cumbrae is a private island; the owners ask for a small donation for visiting the island. *www.weecumbrae.co.uk* Holy Island is the home of the Centre for World Peace and Health; it is accessible to visitors during the day but asks for no overnight camping, so I respected this request and circumnavigated the island instead. *www.holyisle.org*

this journey I had studied tidal flow charts and tide times, planned my route with estimated times and informed the coastguard. I meticulously packed what I needed for one overnight stay and then did it again another time.

I had deliberately left some wriggle room on where to pitch. I wanted to explore and find a good spot that felt right rather than pre-pick everything on a map.

Torrential rain hits just as I'm approaching the bay. It has come early. I get off the water as quickly as possible, the rain washing away my plan of the romanticised photo I had envisaged for entering the bay with its stunning views. I like the authenticity of photography in the wild – nature does not care about your plans!

I chaotically throw all my bags off the board on to the beach, darting around to find cover. Why am I rushing when I know that all my stuff will stay dry, and I have nowhere else to be? Perhaps a deep instinct for survival.

Before long the sun peeks through the clouds and for the rest of the day and night it is glorious! After the early start, I am tired, so I just sit on the island all day long doing not very much except listening to the waves coming in and the birds chirping. I barely see another soul, though a couple of hikers pass who were doing the West Island Way and simply nod from afar. Most of the time people are interested in what you're doing, sometimes remarking on the fact that you're alone, or a woman alone, but mostly with interest rather than judgement.

A seagull sits on a big plastic container going about his day, squawking loudly – a strange sight. In the middle of nowhere on a beautiful beach, this human thing we made looks so out of place in nature and among the wildlife.

Once my energy returns, I start my beach clean. This beach in particular has lots of ghost gear (discarded fishing nets) attached to rocks, so I take out my knife and cut them loose. I feel slightly self-conscious documenting my beach clean, as I would do this anywhere I go, but I remind myself sharing these moments and insights with others and storytelling through photos and videos can go a long way towards raising awareness. I continue up the hill, sometimes looking up and admiring my little red tarp on the beach in the distance. Beach cleaning is of course not the full solution, but looking after my local blue space in this small way leaves me feeling satisfied – it's a two-way relationship.

When I've filled a bag I feel a mix of sadness that this is the reality everywhere, but also that it feels better for taking some – any – positive action, I decide on a quick swim in the sea to help wash away the day. There are little hermit crabs stopping and starting in different homes, and flatfish playing hide and seek under the sand. I marvel at the underwater world, but don't last long in just my swimsuit.

It's time for my evening routine. One of the beautiful things about living here is the opportunity to roam free and camp overnight with just a few exceptions, thanks to the Scottish Outdoor Access Code. It promotes leaving no trace and not overstaying your welcome, but it gives people the chance to connect to nature in a very profound way.

The Kelly Kettle is perhaps not the most obvious choice for carrying around, but I love the authentic feel of heating up water on the fire contained in the little base. My fresh food has been used in the first couple of days, so I am now on to freeze-dried meals. Tonight, it is spinach dhal – it's actually pretty good considering this food was designed for astronauts.

I underestimate how loud the seagulls can be in the night – do they not sleep like we do? I must look that up, I think. A family of ducks also waddle up in a neat row late at night and back in again early in the morning. I feel privileged to witness their little family routine unfold as if I'm not there.

Wrapped up in my sleeping bag and bivvy bag, I am glad that I had practised my tarp set-up in the garden weeks ago. With my headtorch on, I look for a small red drybag, the one marked for my 'evening routine' containing an eye mask, earplugs and, perhaps most importantly, my indulgent bar of chocolate. It's not there. I left it outside my mosquito net in the big drybag next to my board. Shoot! Do I get eaten by Scotland's summer midges but enjoy my evening ritual (and the chocolate), or do I leave it till the morning and have a good night's sleep. Eat or be eaten? I make a run for it. No regrets.

In the middle of the night, I wake once or twice, as I often do, and watch the stars. A reward for sleeping in the open. Sleeping outside seems to have its own currency anyway. How is it I can squeeze into my bivvy bag, sleep for only two hours and still feel amazing waking up in nature, but eight hours in bed is never enough?

The next morning it takes me a while to have my overnight oats for breakfast and pack up, placing everything into dry bags within more dry bags. I somehow never manage to do it exactly the same as the night before, but it all fits fine, and it is time for possibly my favourite moment of any SUP trip.

I jump on my board feeling the weight of the bags, finding my balance again, and take a few strokes in the clear water of the ocean. I am home. It feels good to be on the move again, towards the next island. Everything I need is on my board; I feel full of promise for the day ahead and a freedom that is hard to describe. I imagine it's a bit like bikepacking. A seal pops up in the bay to see me off. I take one last look back at the island and say thank you for having me. I'll never look at it the same way again from the mainland now. I turn and take in the gentle breeze on my face as I set my pace for the next few kilometres.

My family have taken the ferry over to the Isle of Arran and are waiting for me on the beach as I approach Lamlash Bay through the no take zone on my last stretch of water. Lamlash Bay No Take Zone was the first community-led marine reserve of its kind in Scotland when it was established in 2008. No fish or shellfish can be taken from its waters or seabed, including the shore area. It was the result of thirteen years of campaigning by the Community of Arran Seabed Trust.

My daughter runs in for a hug, and my husband – always supportive – is relieved that I arrived as planned.

My daughter sees this as normal; I have always continued my adventures. I think it's okay for her to see that I have my own identity, and I go after what makes me feel alive. My hope is that she will feel free and empowered to do the same. She misses me sometimes, she asks me not to go sometimes and the mum guilt is real, but my cup is full, and I have so much to give again.

Of course, there are also times she will come with me on a calm sunset paddle, and we jump in the water and pootle around the bay until our hands are wrinkly, or she'll sit on my board on an autumn day picking up different colour leaves from the water to make art along the way.

I think it is so important for this generation to build a connection with nature, for their own mental health in busy tech-heavy lives, and to help them see with their own eyes the importance of looking after our planet.

As a volunteer and ambassador for the charity Seaful, which was founded by Cal Major (see page 25), I help run sessions on the Isle of Arran in partnership with the Community of Arran Seabed Trust, taking young people snorkelling and allowing them to experience that marvel for themselves. My hope is that by sharing the beauty of these islands, it will spark an interest in protecting the ocean like it has for me and my daughter.

EXTREME DREAM TO ST KILDA
DEAN DUNBAR

If I stepped one metre either side of where I was standing, I was likely to fall off the cliff and land either in the sea or on a pile of rocks at the foot of the cliff. This remote pile of rocks was potentially very dangerous for a blind person.

The sky is blue, and the wind, well, it's not too bad. Not too bad here in the sheltered bay. There are seventy kilometres of Atlantic Ocean to cross to get to where I want to be, and it's time to go.

But before I tell you about the trip, I need to fill in some bits. I was born in 1969 with full sight. At the age of nine my sight dropped overnight, and I was registered as partially sighted. Seventeen years later my sight took another dip and ever since I have been registered blind. Hey ho, life could always be worse. On the upside, I do have some sight. Did you know that ninety-three per cent of people who are registered blind in the UK do have some sight? It may just be enough to tell whether it is daytime or night, or they may be as lucky as me and be able to make out blurry silhouettes, and occasional movement. So how did I know that the sky was blue, as stated in the opening paragraph? Because Patrick told me! And who is Patrick? Read on.

In 1992, my dad gave me a book called *The Life and Death of St Kilda* by Tom Steel. By the time I had finished reading about the extraordinary group of islands and the amazing life of the people who once lived there, a trip to St Kilda was added to my bucket list. But at that time the only way to get there was as part of a very expensive three-day cruise. As I didn't have a house to remortgage and there wasn't much call for visually impaired bank robbers, the trip would have to wait, for now.

In 1998, I did a tandem skydive, and the adrenaline rush was so intense that this started my love of extreme and adventure sports. Over the next few years, I did all of the usual things: bungee jumping from a helicopter, wing walking, human catapult and adventure racing.

Then in 2008 I met Patrick Winterton. Among his many talents, he is a highly experienced kayaker, having paddled from Scotland to the Faroe Islands and from Shetland to Norway. In 2009, we planned a kayaking trip to St Kilda, a trip he had already done several times, but the weather was against us. Then in 2016, with me now heavily into SUP, I asked him if he would help me SUP to St Kilda, and luckily for me he said 'yes'.

I had already taken on several longer paddles such as the ninety-two-kilometre Caledonian Canal and a fifty-kilometre sea crossing from the Isles of Scilly to Cornwall. On these and many other group paddles, I had had friends paddling with me, acting as sighted guides. I had also done a few solo loch paddles between twenty and forty kilometres in length.

When I paddle solo on lochs, all I am able to see are three layers around me. The bottom layer is white – this is the water on which I'm paddling. The middle layer is black – this is the land that surrounds the loch. The top layer is hopefully light – this is the sky. When paddling on the larger lochs in Scotland, they are generally surrounded by large hills or mountains. These hills run down either side of the loch, and at some point they will meet (normally at the head of the loch), creating a V-shape. The V is my 'sweet spot' that I rely upon. I can't tell if it is one kilometre away or fifty, I just know that that is my target for the day where I hope the end of the loch will be.

There are no sweet spots out at sea, so for this I need a sighted guide. There are only a small number of people I totally trust when on the sea, and Patrick is one of them.

At 5 p.m. on 3 July 2017 we paddled out of the bay at Griminish, on North Uist in the Outer Hebrides. In the bay, there had been some waves, but these were no taller than knee height. Now out of its shelter, the waves were well over head height, and for the next wee while I would be on my knees, trying to spot Patrick in his sea kayak as he vanished behind one wave, only to reappear on the crest of the next one.

For the first two hours it was a real roller-coaster ride, with the difference between the trough and the crest reaching over three metres high. Our goal for this evening was just to get to Haskeir, an island, or rather a pile of rocks, located fifteen kilometres from Griminish. On a flat day I would expect to cover that distance in two hours, but it would take three hours tonight.

Once close to Haskeir, Patrick told me to stay put, while he went to look for a possible landing spot. Left alone for what felt like ages, but was probably no more than ten or fifteen minutes, I stood there listening to the wildlife. There were seals snorting before diving and thousands of seabirds flying from the rocks and diving into the water all around me, some less than a paddle's length away. The frantic flapping of the puffins was very distinct.

People often ask me if my hearing, or my other senses, are much stronger now that I have lost my sight, but I think the answer is 'no'. It's just that I rely on my other senses much more than other people. When I'm walking up the road, I'm constantly tuned in to the traffic on the road and pedestrians on the pavement, listening out for potential obstacles.

It was only now that I started to realise how badly this could go wrong. I'm a blind guy standing on a SUP, fifteen kilometres from North Uist, the closest possible rescue. If something happened to Patrick, firstly how would I know, and secondly what would I do? I ran through all of the potential scenarios, making sure my electronic flare and whistle were still attached to me, and trying to work out which direction I needed to paddle to get back to North Uist.

Then I heard Patrick, and we were off. Because of the volume of the birds calling around us, we swapped from verbal to whistle communications. Patrick blew his whistle, and I paddled towards the sound.

A few minutes later we were in a wee sheltered bay, about the width of a single-car garage, but several storeys high. Sitting in his kayak, Patrick told me that he had spotted a thin ledge about two metres above the water line, and I would need to leap up from my SUP and grab it, where I could then pull myself up and on to Haskeir.

Standing with my board gently bobbing up and down at the foot of the cliff, I leaped up and forward. My hands and upper body hit the cliff wall, and I began to slide down it. It crossed my mind that Patrick may be playing a joke on me, and I was about to slide down the cliff into the water, but no, there it was. My fingertips felt the ledge, I hooked on to it, and I stopped sliding. Hanging there briefly, while I got a better grip, I pulled myself up and bingo, I was on the island. Fifteen minutes later, Patrick, his kayak, my SUP and all of our kit were up there too.

First job was to get out of our wet kit and get something dry and warm on. Next was hot food and something to drink. I was starting to get a bit shaky now. It was nothing to do with temperature or fatigue, it was recognising my lack of input. I was beginning to feel like a passenger on this trip – albeit a passenger who did all of their own paddling – standing there waiting to be fed and looked after.

Since we had arrived on Haskeir, Patrick had pretty much stood me on the only flat piece of rock available, about the size of a front door mat. He had then helped me with my kit, prepared the food and drink, and then sorted everything out. This wasn't some sort of 'control trip' that Patrick was on but was purely done for my safety. If I stepped one metre either side of where I was standing, I was likely to fall off the cliff and land either in the sea or on a pile of rocks at the foot of the cliff. This remote pile of rocks was potentially very dangerous for a blind person. Where were the white lines and handrails? A letter of complaint will be sent.

Joking aside, I did find all of this very hard to deal with. But after a quick chat on the phone with my wife Rhona, I realised that although this standing around being waited on and loss of independence was uncomfortable, it was for my safety, and I was absolutely loving the paddling.

Patrick went off to find a place for us to sleep. Returning a short while later, in the pitch black of the night, he led me further up the cliff to a rock about the size of a football. This was wedged between two sloping rocks either side. He told me I was to sit on this rock and lean back into the narrow gap. He then placed my feet on a smaller rock and told me that this would be my bed for the night, before pinning a tarp above me to shelter me from any rain, and other things that may drop from the sky. He also mentioned that if my feet came off the rock, I would most likely slip off my football seat, and then off the cliff, dropping ten metres or so into the sea below for an early bath. Sweet dreams. He would be sleeping on a narrow edge just a few metres away from me.

As I leaned back into the rocks, I could hear the waves crashing into the other side of the island, less than thirty metres away from me, and the sound of some nesting birds less than a metre away. It was now midnight, and we were planning to be back on the water by 5 a.m. I lay back and thought, *I won't be getting much sleep tonight.* Surprisingly, I slept for about two-and-a-half hours and felt good the next morning.

Back on the water, we launched from the eastern side of the island and paddled around the northern tip to head west. The waves on the western side of the island were almost as big as the previous evening but now there was also the backwash after the waves crashed off Haskeir and came back out again. So, for now, it was back on the knees.

St Kilda was fifty-five kilometres away, but due to the blue sky and sunshine, Patrick was able to see it from Haskeir. Although he had the navigation kit all set up on his kayak, he rarely looked at it.

Over the next ten hours we paddled for fifty-five minutes, rested for five, and started again.

At around ten kilometres from St Kilda, I could make out something on the horizon. Due to my sight issues, the dark blob constantly moved around and disappeared as I moved my head while paddling. It was only when we were about eight kilometres from the giant cliffs (some of the highest sea cliffs in the UK), that the islands became a bit clearer, and I could start using them as a target to aim for. I'm sure Patrick was happy about this, as for the last nine hours, he had been guiding me with the use of a very loud whistle. His ears must have been ringing by now.

At about 3 p.m. on 4 July 2017, we arrived at Village Bay on Hirta, the main island of the St Kilda archipelago.

As I walked ashore, I was covered head to toe in a thick brown crusty layer of salt. This had been caused by ten hours of the wind blowing seawater on to me and then the sun baking it dry. I'm not sure if it was this, or the sight of the tiny wee tent that Patrick and I were due to share, but one of the National Trust for Scotland rangers on the island very kindly invited me to sleep on a bed in the brick-built feather store for the night. Something, they assured me, that was rarely offered to visitors. I very gratefully accepted their sympathy and very kind offer and slept the sleep of a very tired paddler that night. I'll always be grateful to Patrick for his vital help on my paddle to St Kilda.

Since my trip to St Kilda, I have had to adapt my paddleboarding somewhat. After injuring my foot in 2018, which prohibits me from standing up for any length of time, in 2019 I swapped from stand-up paddleboarding to prone paddleboarding. This is where the paddler either kneels or lies down in the prone position, using their hands as paddles. It's hard work, but for me it is much more exhilarating. I know that a lot of people enjoy taking in the view when they SUP, but as a blind paddler, this has never been a thing for me. But lying down, with my face just above the water, listening to the water rush by, or feeling waves crash over my head when on the sea – now that's a full-on sensory delight. I love it!

A HEALING JOURNEY
KATIE SIMMONS

Like a screaming banshee I gave that river my all. This female paddleboarder was firing down world-class rapids and channelling internal strength she thought she had lost.

Before I start, I want you to close your eyes. Take some deep breaths and picture yourself paddling. Surround your senses, feel the paddle in your hands, hear the gentle swoosh of the water as your board moves past the paddle and notice the smell of the air around you. That sense of solitude and freedom is why I fell in love with paddling. The essence of disconnecting from the world and experiencing true wilderness is becoming much harder to find in modern-day society. Paddleboarding opens doors you never thought you were capable of opening.

My name is Katie and I've been lucky enough to have experienced some spectacular and magical places in my life. I come from a working-class background and have built this life around me. It's not been an easy ride and as with most lives it has thrown me multiple lemons that I've had to soften the sour taste off. I work as a professional SUP guide, outdoor instructor and as a nurse in wonderful North Wales. I hope the next few short stories inspire you and fill you with the same warmth I get every time I go paddling.

Knowing where to begin with my story is difficult. I still remember the first time I was invited to paddle on the River Dee at Mile End Mill. A good friend, Ant, had brought some SUPs over from the USA and was launching his business. He needed some wild people to have a go at paddleboarding for a photoshoot. A one-hour photoshoot turned into me being hooked for several hours. It was a new vessel in which I could play on the home rapids! That was thirteen years ago. Since then, I've cried, screamed, smiled, shouted, been silent, been scared, elated and been truly moved while paddling thousands of kilometres across the globe.

By the time SUP was booming in 2018 I had already competed in white-water, flat water and endurance races. As the industry grew, I decided to set sail and raced yachts across the Atlantic. When I returned, I fell in love, but I also fell more deeply in love with the ocean. The weeks spent crossing the Atlantic gave me a thirst to want to do more. So, I started my nursing degree, moved in with a man I had only just met and pursued adventuring further on paddleboards, taking them to places people weren't even aware you could take them. I was setting new standards on inflatable SUPs and multi-day self-supported expeditions.

As this was all so new to me, I dragged my new land-loving partner Tom with me for safety. It took rather a lot of convincing – I had to negotiate thousands of eye rolls and numerous huffs and puffs. He was no stranger to expeditions and had been on numerous ones across the world. However, with me it had to be just that little bit different. I was on a journey of self-discovery and testing my new skills in expedition planning, navigation and rough-water paddling. Tom had only been paddling with me a few times when I suggested our first multi-day paddle around Raasay and Rona. These two islands are sandwiched between the Isle of Skye and the north-west coast of Scotland. For some reason he agreed with my plan and the next day we found ourselves on the dimly lit and cold Sconser slipway with boards and bags packed. In essence, we were ever so slightly winging it.

As midday approached and the tides turned, we left and paddled into the afternoon, a gentle breeze and oscillating waves pushing us a few kilometres along Raasay to camp one. This was a well-planned site with a freshwater stream overlooking the mainland. As the sun began to set, the lapping waves hit the shore coloured in the gentle pinks and purples from the Scottish sky, golden eagles called above us, and a light wind held off the midges. It was all so perfect.

Little did we know what was in store. The next day we awoke to winds stronger than forecasted but still blowing in the correct direction.

We decided to crack on with our day as we headed to the channel in the islands between Raasay and Rona. We had a distance of sixteen kilometres ahead of us to navigate with cliffs and exposed sections of water. As we turned the corner heading toward Fearns, I learned my first major lesson. The fetch – the distance wind travels over water unobstructed and in a constant direction – created by the storm was enormous. Tom and I looked at each other, nodded and pushed forward. Hours later we were both on our knees with loaded boards getting smashed by breaking waves and pushed by a cross-shore wind (the wind blowing parallel to the shoreline). We were battling not to get pushed into the cliffs. At this point it all became a struggle, and I started to think, *What have I done? I'm going to get us hurt, we're going to need rescuing!* I thought I had made a huge mistake.

As exhaustion hit me, I could only imagine how Tom was feeling. Progress was slow if not backwards at times, but as I turned around, he was there battling away saying, 'It's not that bad', laughing his head off at the ridiculous situation we found ourselves in. Meanwhile, I was holding back the desperate tears. As we approached the channel between the islands, the wind broke and we were finally pulled into calm waters. We hauled our boards up on to the rocks and collapsed. But shortly after, our midday nap was interrupted when half the island's population of seals made their appearance. Over one hundred seals were climbing over our boards surrounding us. Tom reckoned they were eyeing up the cheese board.

We left and turned around the island recharged and ready to paddle into the headwind, pushing on looking for the perfect camping spot. At a quick pitstop to top up our water supplies, we met a woman who asked us if we had seen the orca that had just passed her. Suddenly the hasty arrival of all the seals earlier made sense!

The paddle against the wind had made us later than we had planned. With force 4 to 5 winds, we decided to try the channel between Eilean Fladday and Raasay for some shelter. The channel had dried up by the time we arrived, so portage it was. Tom was under strict instructions not to leave our two brand new touring boards alone. As I hobbled with our bags on the seaweed over the ridge and down the other side, Tom appeared with just one board. I immediately shouted, 'The board, Tom! The other board!' The strong wind was funnelling down the gap and as I ran up to the ridge there was my board and paddle blowing away into the sea. Tom was still standing there eating his Penguin bar. I ran down the pebbles and crashed into the sea swimming as fast as I could. Every time I reached to grab the board, I narrowly missed it. Then I felt the sting. A deep burning feeling, something so intense it made me swim even faster almost to the point of exhaustion. Finally, I reached the board. I hauled myself on to it breathing heavily and looked at my new shoulder accessory – a lion's mane jellyfish. It was a small one that had wedged itself between my buoyancy aid, my shoulder and my 0.5-millimetre neoprene wetsuit. Once I reached the shore I shouted and bawled, crying that I hated what we were doing, and it was a stupid idea. Tom, who was still eating his Penguin bar, chuckled and said, 'It's from these experiences that we learn and get better.'

The next morning, we awoke to stillness; even now the memory of this brings me a sense of calm. Mirror-calm waters, deep pinks and purples, otters playing below our campsite. There were dolphins and porpoises breaching next to us for the next section of the journey and we were accompanied by the faint sounds of Gaelic music coming from a local fishing boat. We had done it! I cried and thanked the Scottish gods for giving us such a special morning and thanked Tom for just being him, for taking it all in his stride. He held me in his arms and told me, 'Your passion for this silly sport is unfathomable, Katie. You're going to do great things, and I can't wait to watch this journey and be by your side.'

That was our first expedition together. For the next four years we laughed, learned and cherished all our time spent outside in this incredible world.

Little did I know then how life would turn out. In 2020, Tom and I got engaged after my stint with the Army Reserves as a medic. On 11 June 2022, Tom died, three months before we were due to get married, four days before my final wedding dress fitting and five days before my birthday. My life fell apart in front of me. Tom died as a result of a climbing accident. He was a qualified mountaineering and climbing instructor out on a solo day on a scramble he had done a tonne of times. I knew something was wrong when he stopped checking in at 11 a.m. I finished my shift in A&E at 2 p.m. and went looking for him in the mountains. For over four hours I was frantically searching for his waterproof, a body, a person who had seen him. It wasn't until 7 p.m. that night I was told over the phone alone in a car park opposite Tryfan that he wasn't coming back. The darkness crept in very fast.

Not only had I lost the man I loved more than anything, but over the next year I lost myself. A large part of me died when I lost him, and it continued to die. He was the man who made me believe in myself and without him I was utterly lost.

The guidance from my close network ensured I didn't give up paddleboarding, as much as I wanted to. I had convinced myself that there was nothing left for me in this world and that I should be with Tom. My friends dragged me out on boards, even though I was unwilling to take part. I had taken so much pride in converting the land lover into a paddleboarder that every time I approached the board I would just break down.

Messages would flood into my social media of how much of an inspiration I was for carrying on, how I had impacted paddlers' lives when I was guiding or instructing or simply from just chatting to them. I knew Tom would have been furious if I didn't carry on. So, I did. On the outside I was a highly professional guide, a psyched and passionate young woman leading the way in SUP guiding. On the inside every paddle was painful, every guiding trip a real internal test.

I gradually started to open up about how grief really affects us all, and from then on I started to heal.

I also wanted to test myself. An opportunity presented itself in the shape of the Grand Canyon, a 281-mile descent of the Colorado River with some of the most skilled paddlers I knew. So naturally the answer was 'yes, as long as I can take my paddleboard.' A sixteen-day self-supported trip for eight of us. Two rafts, four kayaks and one paddleboard. I swallowed my fear, embraced Tom's psych and took on the biggest rapids I had ever seen in my life.

Like a screaming banshee I gave that river my all. This female paddleboarder was firing down world-class rapids and channelling internal strength she thought she had lost. My healing journey, a rediscovery of myself, validation of how strong I had become. I had unknowingly become the first British paddleboarder to descend the Colorado River on a SUP.

When you feel so lost, it's not until you're in the middle of an unknown place with unknown consequences that you really find yourself again. I now know why I was sent on that journey. I have since shared my story in a room full of women at the #ShePaddles festival run by Paddle Cymru. A journey I was terrified to tell people about, but there I was in a room full of supportive women, helping to inspire others.

With more paddles planned in the pipeline, I now paddle not only for myself but for Tom. I'm on a constant journey of healing and to help others on their own journeys.

CONTRIBUTORS

STEPH BARNICOAT

At a very young age, Steph had a fascination for the ocean and all creatures inhabiting it, with a big passion for marine mammals. She now works in marine mammal consultancy. Steph loves paddleboarding and being on the water. This led her to becoming a SUP instructor and setting up her own business, SUP with Steph, with her dog, Percy, joining in too. When Steph is not exploring the Cornish coast on her SUP, she and Percy can usually be found walking the South West Coast Path.

Favourite place to paddle: Porthpean in Cornwall. The Scottish lochs are becoming new favourites too.
Favourite piece of kit: my Palm Equipment Atom dry trousers and Percy's Terrain Dog swim vest.
Favourite paddling drink or snack: a vegan Cornish pasty from Philps.
Top SUP tip: if you want to start SUP but feel a little scared or anxious, ignore the fear, book that lesson, join a club and just get out there!

supwithsteph.wixsite.com/website
@steph_and_percy

CONTRIBUTORS

WILL BEHENNA

Will Behenna has been paddleboarding since 2021 and is passionate about enabling everyone, especially those who have difficulty standing, to get out on the water. He has designed and built a range of inclusive paddleboarding equipment and works with coaches and groups across the country supporting them to make their paddleboarding opportunities more accessible. He is constantly pushing the boundaries to see what is possible. If you need any advice or support to help get more people paddling, please get in contact.

Favourite place to paddle: Christchurch Harbour in Dorset.
Favourite piece of kit: my paddleboarding seat.
Favourite paddling drink or snack: sugary tea and cake.
Top SUP tip: always be prepared; have lots of kit for that 'just in case' moment.

www.inclusivepaddleboarding.co.uk
@inclusivepaddleboarding

DAISY BEST

Dr Daisy Best is a counselling psychologist, director of her own independent psychology practice and author of academic papers on trauma. She has been paddleboarding since 2021 and is on a quest to paddleboard every canal in the UK. So far, Daisy has paddled over 650 miles of canals and has raised over £8,000 for Mind in the process. She advocates for the benefits paddleboarding has on mental health. Daisy is one of the volunteer organisers for the annual Paddlefest at Scaling Dam Sailing and Watersports Club in North Yorkshire.

Favourite place to paddle: whenever I see a canal, I do get very excited, and my favourites so far are the Llangollen and the Caledonian. However, my closest canal is around an hour away so my regular place to paddle is the River Esk betweem Ruswarp and Sleights, which I love. In the winter, I am often the only person there – just the herons, ducks and me.

Favourite piece of kit: Legacy Watersports kayak trolley – perfect for towing my SUP when I have to walk around locks on canals. I tie the trolley to the back of my SUP, then flip it over and pull.

Favourite paddling drink or snack: I am vegan so I usually take my own food and snacks as I can't always guarantee that I will be able to locate what I need. I must admit, any vegan 'jelly' sweets are a firm favourite to freshen the palate – I enjoy removing them from my teeth with my tongue when my hands are occupied as I pack my SUP away!

Top SUP tip: never disregard what you are capable of achieving for yourself, on a SUP and in life.

@c2csup2023

CAROLINE DAWSON

Caroline Dawson, or Caz as she's known, is a passionate and skilled stand-up paddleboard coach and guide with an infectious love for adventure. Her award-winning business, SUP Lass Paddle Adventures, is nestled in the heart of the stunning Clwydian Range and Dee Valley National Landscape in North Wales, giving her access to an array of beautiful paddle locations that she eagerly shares with her clients.

Beyond the Welsh countryside, Caz has led thrilling multi-day expeditions across Scandinavia, always aiming to make each adventure not just accessible but unforgettable. Her adventurous spirit is demonstrated by her participation in numerous long-distance and challenging paddle events.

In an awe-inspiring feat, in 2024 Caz became the first woman to stand-up paddleboard over 330 kilometres along the mighty Madre de Dios, a major tributary of the Amazon, during her journey through the Peruvian Amazon.

Favourite place to paddle: the River Dee – my river. It's a place I feel deeply connected to on so many levels. From its source in the Welsh hills to where it meets the sea near Chester, I've paddled nearly every stretch of it. There are parts of the river that feel truly magical and untouched, and every time I'm out there, I feel incredibly fortunate to be able to soak it all in. It's not just the beauty of the river, but the sense of peace it gives me – there's something special about being on the water, breathing in the surrounding nature and feeling like I'm part of the landscape.

Favourite piece of kit: my trusty Kelly Kettle. I actually inherited it from my dad, a well-worn, battered version that had been on countless fishing trips on the River Dee and the west coast of Ireland. By the time it came into my hands, it was at least thirty years old, but it had so many memories attached to it. That old kettle has since retired, replaced with a newer, safer version, but I still love its simplicity. There's something about the Kelly Kettle that always sparks a conversation, gets people involved and delivers the perfect, warming brew. It's an absolute must-have for anyone who loves the outdoors.

Favourite paddling drink or snack: I love to taste the location after a paddle, whether it's indulging in a delicious local Welsh ice cream or enjoying a soft, fluffy Norwegian skoleboller. I'm always on the lookout for the best, most traditional local treats to enjoy – not just for myself, but for my guests too. It really enhances the whole paddling experience and supports the fantastic artisan businesses that make these goodies. There's something about savouring a local snack that makes you feel even more connected to the place you've just explored.

Top SUP tip: be brave enough to suck at something new. We were all beginners once, and trust me, I still remember the days of jelly legs and bird claw feet when I first started. My advice is simple: relax, smile and keep going. Progress comes with time, and I promise you'll get there. There's no one-size-fits-all way to master skills, so don't be afraid to experiment and find your own path. Every attempt, even the wobbly ones, is a step forward!

www.suplass.com
@sup_lass

DEAN DUNBAR

Dean Dunbar was born with full sight. At the age of nine he was registered as partially sighted and at twenty-seven was registered blind. Two years later he got into extreme and adventure sports, taking up SUP in 2014 and prone paddleboarding in 2019. Since 1998, Dean has set twenty-nine world firsts. He also talks about his adventures at public and private events. As he says, 'Come see the blind man play!'

Favourite place to paddle: Loch Awe in Mid Argyll. It's the UK's longest freshwater loch and I have paddled the full length of it several times, both stand-up and prone paddleboarding. It is both beautiful and wild. But beware, the weather can change in an instant, so if you go there, make sure you're well prepared.
Favourite piece of kit: as a blind paddler, I often paddle with a sighted guide, and comms are very important. Carl Sawyer, my friend who got me into SUP, told me about the hands-free Milo™ comms device. This has been a real game changer, allowing me to be several hundred metres away from my guide, but still be safe.
Favourite paddling drink or snack: for most paddlers, the right fuel is all about getting the right amount of protein, carbs and so on. For me it's always been about eating stuff I enjoy. When paddleboarding, my fuel bag consists of cocktail sausages, dodds (cubes) of cheese and jelly babies. Nutritional value, zero; enjoyment factor, off the scale!
Top SUP tip: always keep a little bit in the tank for when things go pear-shaped.

www.extremedreams.co.uk
www.dean-talks.com

JOHN HIBBARD

John truly embodies the concept that life's better by the water. Growing up in South Devon with a passion for the water has led him to a diverse career from being a professional windsurfer to a paddleboarding entrepreneur. Crowned British windsurfing champion in 2007 and BSUPA champion in 2009, John also founded Red Paddle Co in 2008, which has grown into a premier SUP board and equipment brand. John lives by the beach with his family in South Devon.

Favourite place to paddle: Thurlestone, South Devon. On the right day you can paddle over crystal-clear waters, access small, deserted beaches

and even stop at a pub along the way. If you know when and where to look you can also ride some great waves.
Favourite piece of kit: Red Equipment 11′ Compact paddleboard. It packs up small while still being a great board for covering some distance.
Favourite paddling drink or snack: the post-paddle pint!
Top SUP tip: avoid paddling in offshore winds. They are the most challenging conditions you can experience on a SUP. From the beach the water can look flat and inviting, but winds blowing from the beach and out to sea are lethal as they get stronger the further out you go and trying to paddle back against them is extremely difficult.

@redequipment

SIMON HUTCHINSON

Simon Hutchinson is a dedicated all-season paddler and the host of the SUPfm podcast – the world's leading stand-up paddleboarding podcast.

In the show, Simon connects paddlers at all levels of experience, providing expert insights, inspiring stories and global perspectives on the sport and the water. Covering adventure, racing, surfing, safety and the mental and physical benefits of SUP, the podcast helps listeners to maximise their personal time on the water and to take their paddleboarding journey to the next level.

The SUPfm podcast is available on all podcast platforms.

Favourite place to paddle: Avon Beach in Dorset.
Favourite piece of kit: my Starboard Generation paddleboard.
Favourite paddling drink or snack: a bacon sandwich with red sauce.
Top SUP tip: if you're not getting wetter, you're not getting better.

www.supfmpodcast.com
@supfmpodcast

SCOTT 'SKIP' INNES

Scott 'Skip' Innes is a British endurance paddler and adventurer, best known for winning the SUP category of the 2023 Yukon 1000 – the world's longest unsupported paddle race.

Skip's approach to SUP emphasises adventure over competition. He values the experience of pushing personal boundaries and exploring the wilderness.

Beyond his paddling achievements, Skip is committed to inspiring others. This philosophy is highlighted in his professional career; he is the founder of The SHAC (The Surrey Hills Adventure Company), created to encourage people to get outdoors and challenge themselves, however big the challenge.

Favourite place to paddle: Scotland. It's like a mini-Yukon – it can throw it all at you!
Favourite piece of kit: Yster 17'3" adventure paddleboard and Mustang Survival Torrens thermal jacket.
Favourite paddling drink or snack: during a paddle I like a banana. Post-paddle it has to be a beer.
Top SUP tip: get some advice or lessons from a professional and ask questions of local paddlers when you go somewhere new to explore.

www.theshac.co.uk
@skipattheshac

EMILY KING

Emily King is a world-ranked SUP endurance athlete with over a decade of elite racing experience. She has been the GBSUP technical champion in the 12'6" category six times and is world number one ultra-distance SUP champion. A former surfer, she now competes across oceans, lakes, rivers and even white-water, winning national white-water events. Emily completed the first non-stop circumnavigation of the Isle of Wight on a SUP and was the first SUP paddler to undertake the famous Devizes to Westminster Race. Based in the Gower, she is SUP lead for Paddle Cymru and runs Emily King Coaching, which focuses on physical and mindfulness well-being.

Favourite place to paddle: anywhere in sunshine! Realistically, at home on the Gower in South Wales.
Favourite piece of kit: my Starboard All Star race board and Oscar Propulsion paddle.
Favourite paddling drink or snack: coffee and a toasted teacake at Verdi's Cafe at Mumbles, Swansea Bay.
Top SUP tip: every paddle is worth it, even if it's only for ten minutes.

www.emilykingcoaching.com
@emilykingsup

ANNA LITTLE

Anna Little is the co-founder of the Northern SUP Race Club, a dedicated community for paddleboard racers. A passionate competitor, she races across the UK and recently claimed the title of world sprint champion in the over-fifties women category at the 2024 International Canoe Federation (ICF) SUP World Championships. With years of experience as an exercise specialist, Anna runs her own business, helping people of all ages and abilities achieve their fitness goals. When she's not coaching or racing, Anna is a proud mum of three active boys, balancing family life with her love for adventure and competition.

Favourite place to paddle: any of the lakes in the Lake District.
Favourite piece of kit: SIC RS 14.0 21.5" hard board – it is fast, looks good and takes me on great adventures.
Favourite paddling drink or snack: nuts.
Top SUP tip: work on your all-round fitness as well as paddling – it gets you strong!

www.annalittle.co.uk
@northernsupraceteam
@annalittle.fitness.sup

JAMES LITTLE

James Little is a dedicated member of the Northern SUP Race Team (within the Northern SUP Race Club), competing in races all over the world. Passionate about all things water sports, he has a particular love for foiling and kitesurfing, constantly seeking the thrill of being in the sea. When not racing or riding the waves, he's working as an apprentice electrician and gaining valuable skills in the trade. During the summer months, he also works for KA Adventure Sports, a local water sports centre in Northumberland, where he shares his expertise and love for outdoor adventure. Always on the move, James embodies the perfect mix of athleticism, skill and adventure.

Favourite place to paddle: Beadnell, Northumberland.
Favourite piece of kit: Black Project sprint paddle.
Favourite paddling drink or snack: chocolate.
Top SUP tip: just keep paddling.

@jameslittle06

LEEANNE MACKAY

Leeanne runs her mobile SUP school, Paddle Bliss Nairn, around the Highlands and Morayshire in Scotland. She takes her paddlers to some of the most idyllic paddle spots to ensure they have a positive experience fully embracing all that nature has to offer while learning about vital safety considerations along with paddle skills and techniques. Leeanne co-founded the charity Blue Space Highland to support individuals to access free wellness sessions to enhance their mental health. Her aspiration is to reach as many people as possible to show them a new way to wellness: *water for wellness*.

Favourite place to paddle: this has got to be Nairn on the Moray Firth in Scotland. It has three gorgeous sandy beaches, all filled with so much to see from the sea. I often come across playful seals and dolphins, knots (a member of the sandpiper family) playing hide and seek, and experience a whole new perspective on life by seeing the land from the water.

Favourite piece of kit: my Yak Kallista buoyancy aid. It's very well made and fitted, not too bulky so it doesn't hinder me when I need to clamber back on to my board and, at 50N buoyancy, I feel very safe when in the water. It's an added layer so it keeps me warmer in wintertime too.
Favourite paddling drink or snack: I love to make a nice cappuccino at home to take with me on my paddles and I enjoy a piece of lemon drizzle cake too.
Top SUP tip: to live fully in the moment while out on your paddle adventure use *Right Now*, one of The Decider skills (*www.thedecider.org.uk*). To try this, notice five things you can see, four things you can hear, three things you can touch, two things you can smell and take one slow deep breath. Doing this will help you experience complete mindfulness in nature.

paddleblissnairn.co.uk
www.bluespacehighland.org
@paddleblissnairn
@bluespacehighland

CAL MAJOR

Cal Major is an ocean advocate, world-record adventurer and veterinary surgeon. She has undertaken numerous paddleboarding expeditions as a vehicle to discuss important ocean conservation subjects, including being the first person to paddleboard from Land's End to John o' Groats, and circumnavigating Scotland. She has produced and presented award-winning films, and was awarded the prime minister's Points of Light award for her work. She founded the charity Seaful to connect more people to our ocean and inspire stewardship.

Favourite place to paddle: anywhere in my favourite country in the world, Scotland. World-class ocean wildlife, scenery, camping and exciting adventures – there's so much variety, and the conditions are often challenging, which makes it even more special when you have a wonderful adventure, big or small.
Favourite piece of kit: Palm Equipment Atom dry trousers or Fuse

drysuit – these have been total game changers for paddling year-round, especially in Scotland.
Favourite paddling drink or snack: a massive slab of cake.
Top SUP tip: this is a tough one as there have been so many lessons! I think respect for the ocean is the most important though. Don't take a forecast as a given, and don't ever expect to be stronger than the sea. You're always stronger than you think, but the ocean is always stronger than you. So don't get cocky or complacent – work with the ocean not against her, respect her power and always consider what you'll do if the conditions change without warning.

www.calmajor.com
www.seaful.org.uk
@cal_major
@seafulcharity

KATHY MARSTON

Kathy Marston is the founder of Happiest When Outdoors, where she blends her love for movement, nature and well-being through yoga, paddleboarding and adventure. With over ten years of yoga teaching experience, she specialises in SUP yoga, offering unique sessions on the water that bring balance, strength and connection to nature. Passionate about outdoor living, she encourages others to embrace movement in the elements, finding freedom and peace through breath, flow and exploration.

Favourite place to paddle: Derwent Water in the Lake District. Every paddle is different due to the weather and seasons.
Favourite piece of kit: a Buff neck warmer for winter paddles. Call me crazy, but a warm neck makes all the difference to the number of layers needed!
Favourite paddling drink or snack: chocolate-coated peanuts – good for energy and they don't melt as easily as chocolate does on its own.
Top SUP tip: keep a log of your paddles. What the weather was like, mileage paddled and speed and height of the river. This log is invaluable

at building up your own reference points to more accurately assess conditions before venturing out.

@happiestwhenoutdoors

DALE MEARS

Dale Mears is the founder of the Instagram community Stand Up Paddle UK. He is a trust director of design and technology in secondary schools with a passion for the outdoors and adventure. Dale is a FatStick Boards ambassador and works with many other brands. His background in kayaking has taken him around the world and led him to transitioning to SUP. He is now a dad of three girls and on a quest to share his love for the outdoors with them and encourage other parents to get their kids out on the water safely. He is a regular contributor to *Paddler Magazine* and *SUP Mag UK*, where you can usually find him in the review pages.

Favourite place to paddle: Loch Katrine in the Scottish Highlands – a true place of beauty.
Favourite piece of kit: Palm Equipment Solo Vest PFD – I love it, it is super streamlined and very comfortable.
Favourite paddling drink or snack: Nothing beats a bag of Haribo for a quick fix on the water, or if it's after the session an ice cream goes down a treat.
Top SUP tip: reach out to local paddleboarders for their expertise and local knowledge.

@supwithdale
@standuppaddleuk

CATHY MILES

Cathy Miles had brain surgery following a haemorrhagic stroke in July 2017 that left her paralysed on her right-hand side. She has worked really hard to get back to where she was physically before her stroke and is proud to say she is currently about eighty per cent there.

Adventurer and author Fiona Quinn was Cathy's inspiration to give paddleboarding a go and she hasn't looked back since. She has had some fantastic trips both in this country and abroad.

Favourite place to paddle: Bewl Water in the South East. It has its own microclimate – I always check the weather before heading off but sometimes it changes in the twenty minutes it takes me to get there!
Favourite piece of kit: my Starboard paddleboard. At eleven-and-a-half feet long it is so manoeuvrable – I can turn it on a sixpence and, best of all, it's pink! I also love my Starboard one-piece paddle; it is really light.
Favourite paddling drink or snack: home-made carrot cake with cream cheese frosting.
Top SUP tip: if you're just starting your SUP journey try lots of different instructors. They all explain things in a slightly different way, and one will explain something in a way that instantly makes sense. You may then need a different instructor to explain a different point.

@the_disabled_paddler

ADYA MISRA

Adya Misra is a Paddle UK paddle sports coach (kayak, canoe and SUP), founder of People of Colour Paddle and stand-up paddleboarding coordinator at Liverpool Canoe Club, where she volunteers her time and coaches kayaking, rolling, canoeing and paddleboarding. She has been paddling for over ten years, but continues to stay curious about learning and developing her craft as she embodies her coaching philosophy of curiosity, confidence and resilience. Adya regularly paddles on the sea, rivers and big lakes, while continuing to coach in sheltered waters.

Favourite place to paddle: southern coast of Crete.
Favourite piece of kit: NRS Long Jane style wetsuit.
Favourite paddling drink or snack: black coffee.
Top SUP tip: always wear shoes and a wetsuit while boarding in the UK, regardless of the weather. It's a game changer for skills practice!

@queenadya

CONTRIBUTORS

CLARE OSBORN

Clare Osborn is a nature facilitator, retreat host, event coordinator and passionate ocean advocate. As well as teaching SUP, Clare is certified in various forms of coaching, including Blue Health Coaching™, neuro-linguistic programming, mindfulness and Climate Change Coaching™. The holistic knowledge she has gained enables her to support clients and colleagues with empathy, understanding and deep connection. Clare is passionate about connecting people and wild spaces to inspire stewardship of the ecosystem we are part of. Clare also works as a freelance Carbon Literacy® trainer with the charity POW UK.

Favourite place to paddle: for me, having one place to regularly paddle is like having a mindful sit-spot practice. You can watch as the seasons change, the local wildlife evolves, and you really feel like you are part of that place which in turn I think makes you want to care for it more. The place I teach on the River Wey in Godalming gives this to me. I never bore of it even though it's relatively safe enclosed water – partly canal and partly river – and not far from London. But I love the deep understanding it has given me. From watching the ducklings in spring and counting how many make it, to understanding when the water is too fast, or the river is in flood in the winter. It reminds me that nature will do what it wants and is not at our beck and call.
Favourite piece of kit: I'm really not a gadget/kit person but I stand by Palm Equipment as my go-to for safety gear and clothing. I always take my Sea Soul Blessings cards, created by Pippa Best, with me for a paddle as the quiet and stillness I get on the water gives me the brain space I need for personal reflection. They are a wonderful but simple tool for self-compassion and fit easily in my waterproof bumbag.
Favourite paddling drink or snack: pre-paddle it has to be coffee – in a flask or iced in summer. I am powered by it, until I'm not. Post-paddle is usually whatever cereal bar hasn't yet been consumed that is hiding, usually squashed, at the bottom of my dry bag.
Top SUP tip: always anchor your clients when leading mindfulness on the water. Otherwise, they scatter like ducklings and are more focused on that than relaxation.

CONTRIBUTORS

www.clareosborn.com
@wild_ocean_soul

GEMMA PALMER-DIGHTON

A passionate paddleboarder based in Cambridgeshire, Gemma Palmer-Dighton finds boundless joy and challenge on the UK's waterways, from the serene River Great Ouse to the majestic lochs of Scotland. Her journey, sparked by a love for micro-adventures and a desire to explore, has evolved from wobbly beginnings to racing and multi-day camp-out trips. Currently working towards a paddle sports qualification, she is also a Paddle UK #ShePaddles ambassador, championing diversity and aiming to make paddleboarding accessible to all.

Keen for a paddle? Get in touch!

Follow her year-round adventures on Instagram – pushing her limits in racing and training through the darker months, then embracing playful exploration on the waterways as the weather warms and the days lengthen.

Favourite place to paddle: no contest – the majestic lochs and the serene canals that weave through the Great Glen in Scotland. And Loch Ness? Simply unforgettable. You have to experience its beauty for yourself.
Favourite piece of kit: it has to be my Gill women's Verso drysuit or my Gill women's Pursuit neoprene leggings. They're my elemental armour – essential for staying comfy, especially if a beach launch is on the cards.
Favourite paddling drink or snack: elderflower cordial made up with chilled sparkling water served on ice garnished with cucumber and strawberry. Refreshing, floral and utterly delicious.
Top SUP tip: waterside or in camp, turn your board upside down (fin up) – this protects the fin, stops the wind flipping your board and your board becomes a handy seat.

@getgemma

CONTRIBUTORS

HEATHER PEACOCK

Heather lives in Tynemouth, in the north-east of England, with her husband and two children. She discovered paddleboarding in 2007 in Maui where she caught her first wave and has been hooked ever since. Her journey has led her to become an instructor, a water safety advocate and a volunteer for her local coastguard rescue team – the Tynemouth Volunteer Life Brigade. She loves any opportunity to get in the water and to share her knowledge with others.

Favourite place to paddle: Bamburgh in Northumberland – the views are simply magnificent, with its huge castle rising up out of the sand dunes and miles of white sandy beach.
Favourite piece of kit: my custom SMIK SUP surfboard. The dimensions were made especially to my specification, and the aesthetic design is my own. It has transformed my surf experience, and I love the colours of it in the water.
Favourite paddling drink or snack: it's always cake. Any cake will do!
Top SUP tip: my best piece of advice would be to learn about the conditions you're going in to. Being able to understand what the sea is doing and why is a key skill for both staying safe, and maximising the amount of fun you can have. Catching waves is so much fun, you just need to know your limits and understanding the conditions is a key part of this. If you're not sure about the conditions, don't risk going in – ask at your local surf shop or look at trusted web sources like the RNLI and Surfing England to find out more.

@heatherpea

BRENDON PRINCE

Brendon Prince is a world-record-holding stand-up paddleboarder, ex-teacher, lifeguard and water-safety crusader who has swapped the classroom for coastlines. He's passionate about water safety, drowning prevention, extreme SUP adventures and making the English Riviera the go-to destination for all things paddle-powered. Whether he's planning epic events such as the 2026 ICF SUP World Cup: English Riviera or training for No Land, No Limits – a world record attempt to paddle 500 kilometres non-stop – his work is all about safer waters and stronger communities.

Favourite place to paddle: having visited *every* beach and headland around the UK coastline, this is a tough question. My top twenty are for myself and myself alone – coming in at twenty-one is the stretch of the Northumberland coast from Sugar Sands (near Longhoughton) to Alnmouth. Make sure you understand winds and tidal flow before attempting this almost-ten-kilometre paddle.
Favourite piece of kit: my paddle – I'm a Blackfish team paddler. Your paddle is the piece of kit that you use more than anything else; make sure it is perfect for your ability, style of paddling and stature. Get your paddle right and your paddling becomes effortless.
Favourite paddling drink or snack: before and during a paddle, it's water; after a paddle, it's cider. Hydration must be your friend when paddling long distances, especially in an environment that literally sucks the water from you. But once I'm off the water, nothing beats a cold South Devon cider.
Top SUP tip: get the right fin for your paddling. Your fin has a major impact on the ride you'll experience; use the wrong-shaped fin for the conditions and you are in for a bumpy ride. The fin is the 'forgotten' reason why you keep falling off your board. Pay good money for the right fin and you will thank me, hopefully by buying me a cider!

www.brendonprince.com
www.abovewater.org
@brendonprincesup
@abovewateruk

SHILPA RASAIAH

Shilpa Rasaiah undertook her first adventure quite late in life, having never done anything like this before. Aged nearly sixty, she paddled the length of the Grand Union Canal, some 170 miles, showing herself that you are never too old to go on an adventure! In 2024, Shilpa became an Ordnance Survey Champion, which has further pushed her personal boundaries to go on camping and trekking adventures exploring new places to paddle. She has rediscovered her love for the outdoors in much later life. Her latest outdoor 'venture' is taking on an allotment jointly with a friend and finding immense pleasure in very simple things like watching vegetables grow and being in such a wonderful tranquil space.

Favourite place to paddle: I love paddling on long journeys and camping along the way close to the water, where I am able to 'sleep, paddle, eat and repeat' without having to get into a car. I carry everything I need on my touring SUP board.
Favourite piece of kit: my 13' Quroc Allwater paddleboard. It is great in choppy conditions, super stable and it has lots of practical bungees and handles which allow me to easily load my camping gear on to it.
Favourite paddling drink or snack: a hot cup of spicy Indian chai, served in my beautiful floral Japanese design mug that keeps it piping hot for ages.
Top SUP tip: go on an adventure that pushes your personal comfort zone. Don't be afraid to adapt it to make it work for you – it could transform your life.

@Shilpa_Outdoors

CRAIG SAWYER

Craig Sawyer is a UK-based ultra-endurance paddler, personal trainer and film-maker. With over two decades in water sports, he specialises in ultra-endurance SUP racing and multi-day expeditions. Passionate about pushing limits, Craig inspires others to take on challenges that break past self-imposed boundaries.

Favourite place to paddle: the River Arun in Sussex – it's my regular stomping ground for distance training; you can do around sixty kilometres. It's massively affected by the tides so takes planning to get it right; I don't recommend it for beginners. From passing underneath Arundel Castle, gliding past Amberley chalk pits and spotting the infamous Kevin the seal, every time I paddle on the Arun it throws up something different.

Favourite piece of kit: Mustang Survival Greenwater dry bags. These bulletproof bags will outlast me. A top zip with no need to roll down to seal makes it really easy to access the contents and its square shape sits perfectly on the board.
Favourite paddling drink or snack: it would be too obvious to talk about sport-specific nutrition but one of my favourite paddle treats is a Soreen malt loaf snack pack.
Top SUP tip: it sounds cheesy, but we truly are more capable than we give ourselves credit for – seek what's beyond your comfort zone and you'll find a whole new incredible world.

www.thesupcoach.co.uk
@craigsawyer77

KATIE SIMMONS

Katie in a nutshell: a woman who's been through a fair few things in her short thirty-one years. Always connected to the outdoor environment, growing up as an only child on a smallholding she saw nature as a brother or sister. She always had a deep obsession with the sea and marine life and that's something that has continued into her adult years and into her professional work as a freelance outdoor instructor and SUP guide. Being out on the sea she finds a deep sense of feeling at home. Katie is the founder of the Tom Furey Memorial Trust, an ambassador for Palm Equipment and a rep for Surfers Against Sewage.

Favourite place to paddle: I've been super lucky to have paddled in some incredible places around the world, but every time I paddle on the west coast of Scotland just a little bit of my heart always gets left behind there. It's starting to become a second home; I love the beauty and the fact that every day is just so different there. And of course, it's the wildlife that really pulls me back every time.
Favourite piece of kit: this is a hard one, I am a self-confessed kit geek but also someone who's incredibly sensitive to kit, so everything has to be right. My trusty O'Shea 12'6" GTS board has carried me thousands of miles and every other board I have paddled has never really matched up to it. It skips over waves, moves fast and of course it's lightweight and

durable for expeditions. Highly recommended! A close second would be my Palm Equipment Quick SUP belt – it's less faff due to the design, works super well and it's safe.

Favourite paddling drink or snack: this has changed over the years; however, anyone who's paddled with me will know there is always either a Penguin bar or a Tunnock's caramel wafer (another nod to Scotland) in my buoyancy aid pocket. Albeit it is sometimes slightly soggy with added sea salt for flavour!

Top SUP tip: fall off, fall off lots! Or jump, step or slide off your board. Before I head out on some of my hard paddles, I always look at the worst case scenario. I always dress for a potential dip into the water but knowing I can get back on to my island of safety in all conditions is super important. I meet lots of people who are too worried to fall in because they are unsure if they'll be able to rescue themselves – this is one of the most important skills you will learn. Go and get wet – play in those slightly challenging environments with someone. It's here that you'll learn the most about yourself.

@katiethesupnurse
www.tomfureymt.org

MELODY SMITH

Melody, a passionate nature-loving outdoor enthusiast and proud mother and grandmother, has triumphed over breast cancer, emerging stronger and more positive. Through her journey, she discovered the transformative power of paddleboarding, using it as a way to reconnect with nature, find peace on the water and strengthen both body and mind.

Passionate about sharing her experience, she advocates for the benefits of positivity and resilience, inspiring others to embrace the outdoors and experience the healing benefits of being in nature, empowering them to boost their mental health and maintain a positive outlook on life too.

Now working in a demanding role as a team leader in the ambulance service, she finds her time on the water to be more essential than ever. Paddleboarding provides a much-needed escape, helping her reset, recharge and maintain balance in both body and mind, embracing the restorative power of water.

Favourite place to paddle: this is a difficult one to answer. Ideally, I want the perfect balance of sun, sea, sand and play. On a perfect day at low tide (and not after a storm) I love nothing better than to paddle over to the sandbar at Hayling Island in Hampshire, play about on the board in the shallows, stop for a board picnic on the 'desert island' sandbar and soak in the tranquillity and beauty around me.
Favourite piece of kit: my large Jobe drybag. I'm known among my paddle pals for being the one who packs for every eventuality and always brings a picnic! My Jobe bag fits it all and is easy to sling over my back when portaging.
Favourite paddling drink or snack: while I do always pack a snack and drink, I will admit that many of our paddles are planned around a pub stop. On a glorious summer's day nothing beats a drink and chunky chips!
Top SUP tip: don't be afraid of falling in. It means you have that much more practice at being able to self-rescue, which is essential. Always pack spare clothing for those non-summer paddles.

@supositivity

SARAH THORNELY

Also known as SUPJunkie, Sarah lives in Hampshire with her husband and has two wonderful, very grown-up children. SUP came into and transformed her life in 2012 and since then it has been a beautiful rollercoaster of learning new skills, meeting wonderful people and travelling the world. The joy it has brought her over these years has been immense, taking up almost every waking moment of her life and she would not be without it.

Favourite place to paddle: the River Wey is so beautiful and meanders through three English counties.
Favourite piece of kit: my Red Equipment waterproof dry pouch comes on every trip.

Favourite paddling drink or snack: a good strong coffee and slice of cake.
Top SUP tip: keep your mind open to constantly learning new SUP skills.

www.supjunkie.co.uk
@supjunkie.uk

LINN VAN DER ZANDEN

Linn is a paddleboarding guide, expedition host for adventure companies, photographer and speaker. She is passionate about ocean protection, conservation and working with women and young people to build a connection with nature. Linn enjoys multi-day SUP adventures, surfing, sailing, snorkelling and adventures with purpose. She also volunteers with various ocean-centred charities to help make a difference on her doorstep. She lives in the south-west of Scotland with her family.

Favourite place to paddle: my local coastline and surrounding islands in the south-west of Scotland. Seamill Beach is a great place for accessible entry and has a great view of the Isle of Arran for a sunset.
Favourite piece of kit: the Palm Equipment women's dry pant – they are waterproof with attached feet, so you can walk into the water and keep warm all year round.
Favourite paddling drink or snack: I love to make a hot cup of tea with my Kelly Kettle along the way.
Top SUP tip: your ability to live outside your comfort zone on an adventure is much higher than you think. You can do hard things, make hard decisions and bring ideas that seem difficult at first to life if you plan, prepare and you have a desire to make it happen.

@microadventuregirl

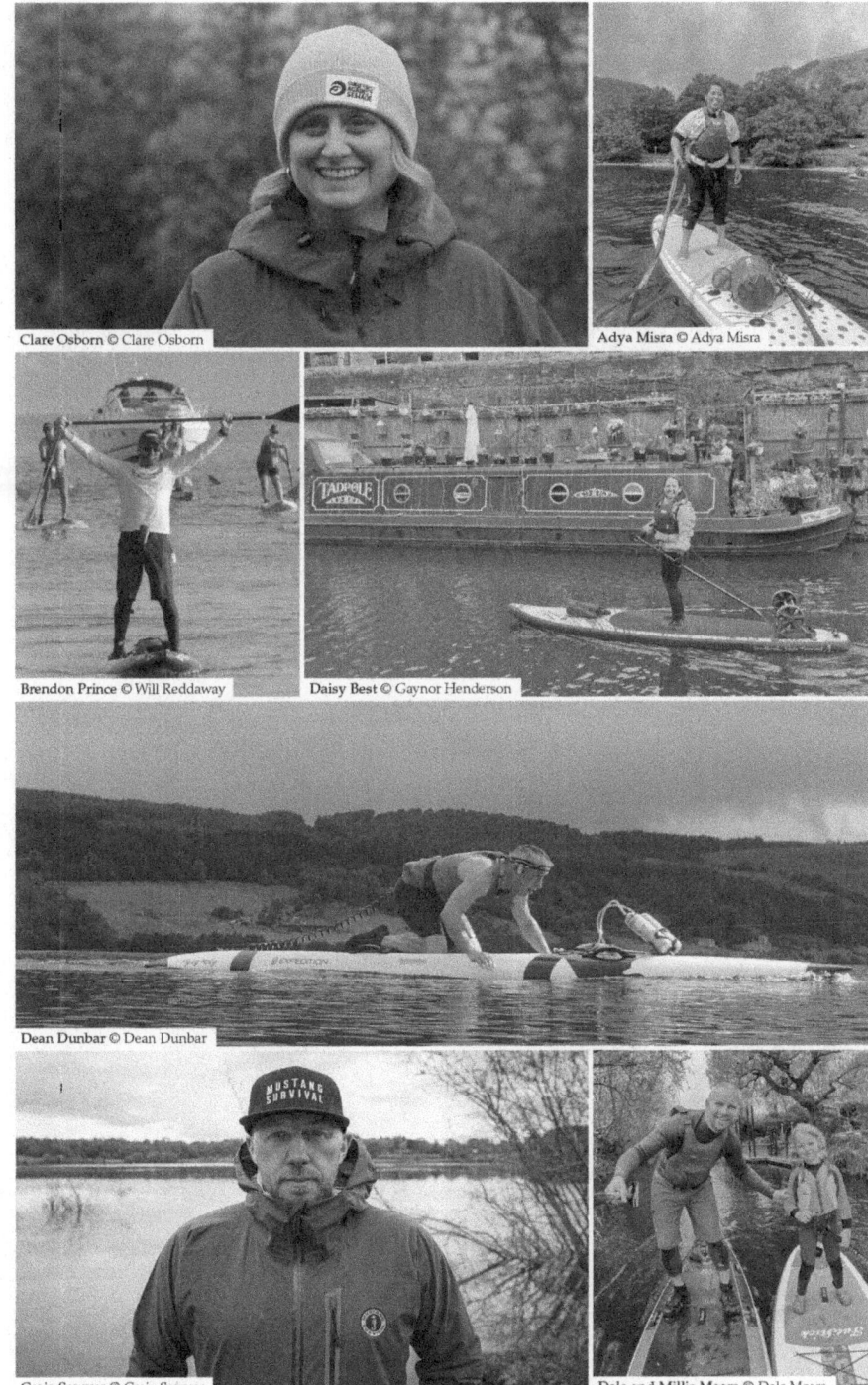

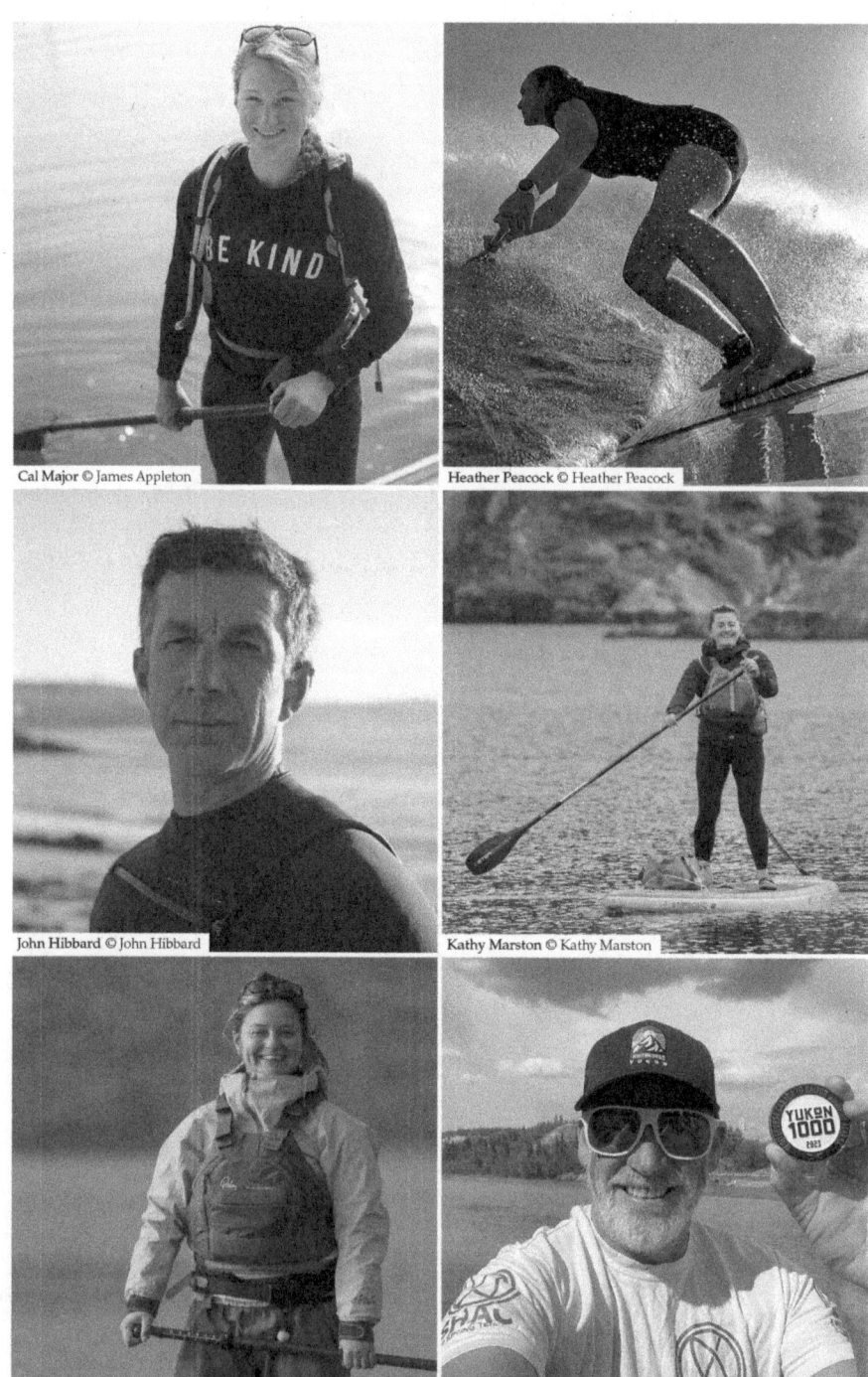

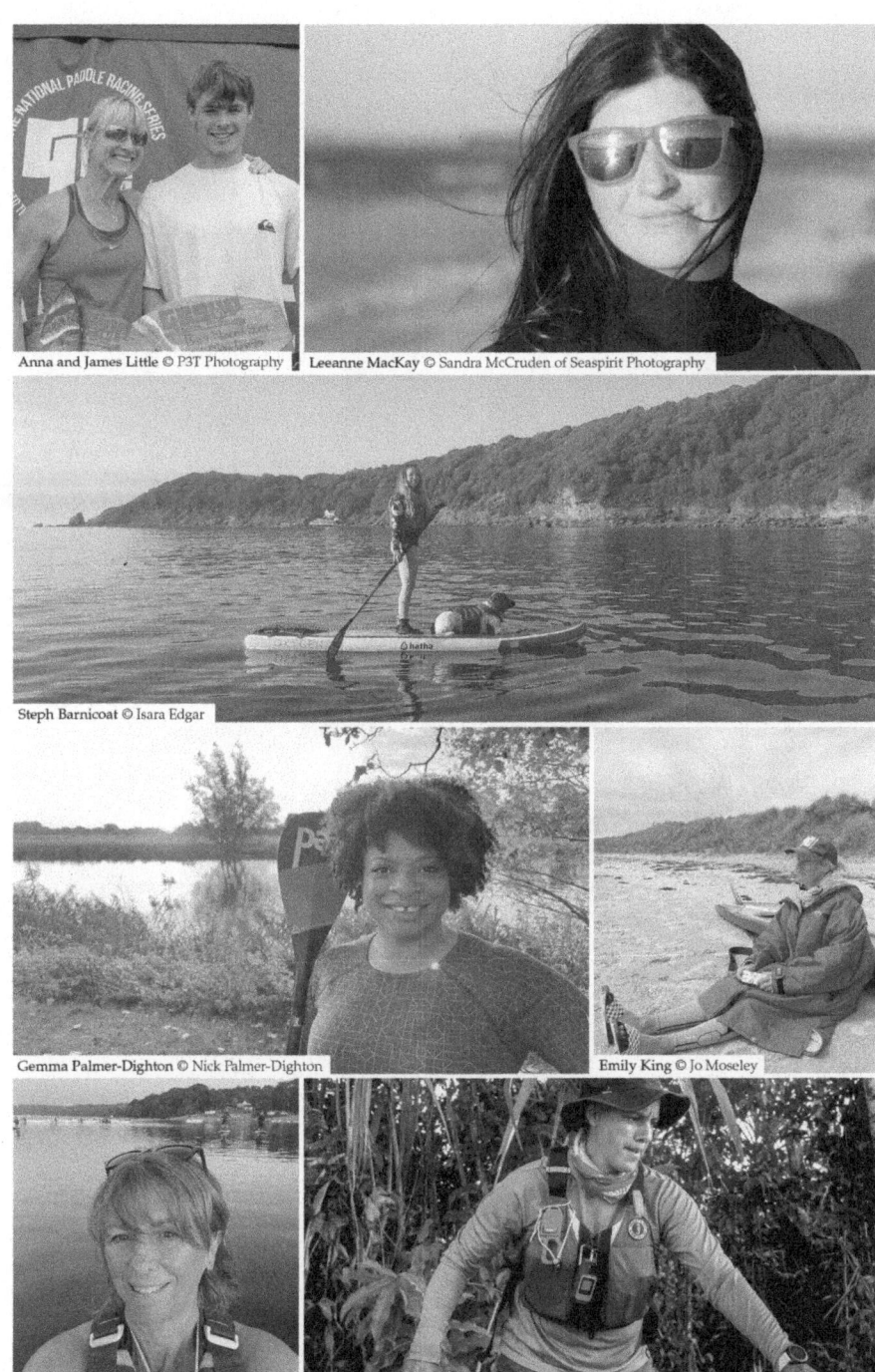

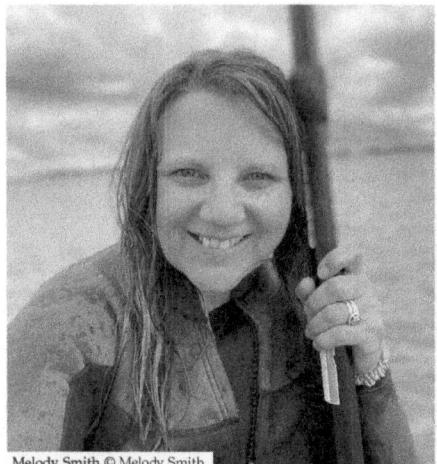
Melody Smith © Melody Smith

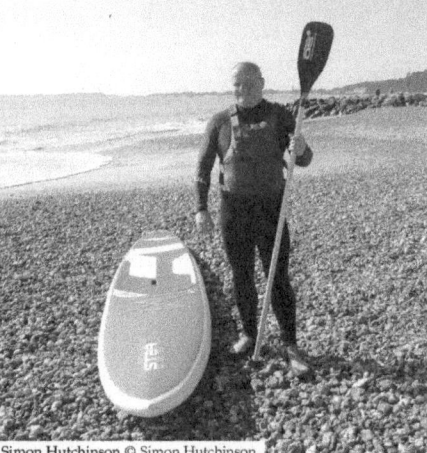
Simon Hutchinson © Simon Hutchinson

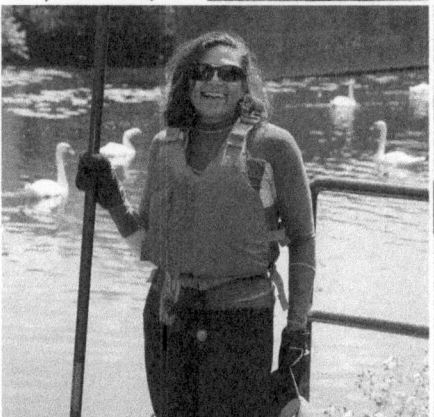
Shilpa Rasaiah © Simon Higginson

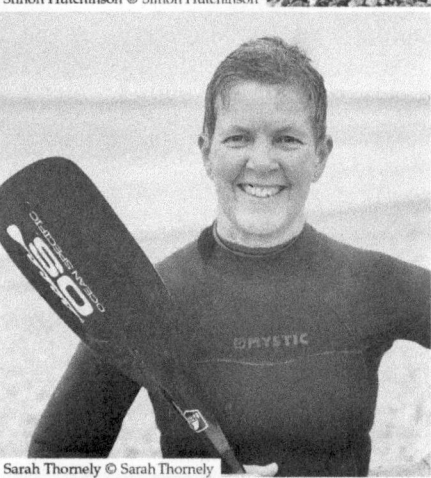
Sarah Thornely © Sarah Thornely

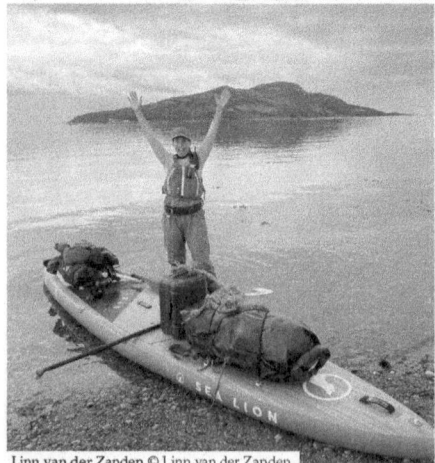
Linn van der Zanden © Linn van der Zanden

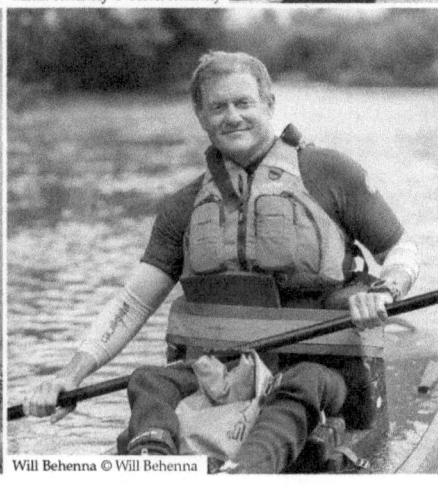
Will Behenna © Will Behenna

ABOUT THE EDITOR

Jo Moseley came to stand-up paddleboarding (SUP) in her early fifties as a way to heal her knee after an injury. From the moment she stood on a paddleboard on Derwent Water in the Lake District on 24 September 2016, she fell in love. For the first time in a long time, she felt 'like a warrior not a worrier'. In 2019, she became the first woman to paddleboard coast-to-coast, 162 miles along the Leeds and Liverpool Canal and the Aire & Calder Navigation, picking up litter and raising money for the 2 Minute Foundation and The Wave Project. A film about her adventure, *Brave Enough – A Journey Home to Joy* by award-winning Frit Tam of Frit Films, has been screened at prestigious adventure festivals including the Kendal Mountain Festival, Keswick Mountain Festival and Shextreme.

Jo has written two best-selling books: *Stand-up Paddleboarding in Great Britain* (2022) and *Stand-up Paddleboarding in the Lake District* (2024) which won the Lakeland Book Awards Zeffirellis Prize for Guides and Places 2025. A single mum of two grown-up sons, she lives on the Yorkshire Coast. She loves sea swimming and paddleboarding at sunrise and does a daily 2 Minute Beach Clean. She is an Ordnance Survey Champion and an ambassador for Seaful.

Favourite place to paddle: Runswick Bay in North Yorkshire, or the Lake District.
Favourite piece of kit: my Palm Equipment Tika PFD and my Red Equipment changing robe.

ABOUT THE EDITOR

Favourite paddling drink or snack: home-made bliss balls, or a Real-Meal Cacao and Peanut Butter bar, and a flask of decaf Yorkshire Tea. **Top SUP tip:** if you're a beginner, have a lesson with a qualified SUP instructor.

www.jomoseley.com
@jomoseley

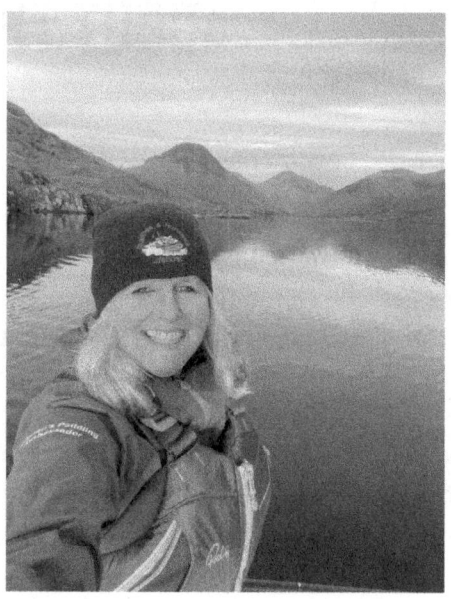

TOP TIPS

- Invest in a lesson or a course of lessons with a qualified instructor.
- Dress for the water temperature, not the air temperature.
- Always wear a buoyancy aid.
- Wear the appropriate leash for the body of water you are on: *www.paddleuk.org.uk*
- Keep your fully charged mobile phone inside a waterproof case on your person, not on your board.
- Plan your paddle in advance. Learn about the location, potential hazards, and entry and exit points.
- Check and know how to understand wind forecasts.
- Some recommendations on maximum wind speeds to paddle in: beginners should aim for a maximum of three miles per hour; when you have a bit more experience, winds of six–eight miles per hour are okay; consider ten miles per hour as the maximum wind speed to paddle in.
- Don't go out in offshore winds – where the wind is blowing from the land out to sea or from the lake shore to the middle of a lake.
- Don't go out in conditions beyond your capability.
- Learn about tides, currents and river conditions and how they impact your paddle.

TOP TIPS

- Have a *float plan*: tell someone where you are going, when you will be back, what to do if you are delayed and when you are safely off the water.
- Go with a responsible friend or group so you can help each other if a problem arises.
- Choose SUP social groups wisely. I recommend going with a group where there are qualified instructors who are taking responsibility for the trip. SUP Yorkshire is a great example.
- Practise self-rescue (how to get back on your board when you fall in).
- Follow specific guidance on kit and safety for SUP surf and white-water SUP.
- To paddle on most rivers and canals in England and Wales you will need a waterways licence. This is included within your Paddle UK membership: *www.paddleuk.org.uk*
- In Scotland you do not need a licence to paddleboard due to the Land Reform (Scotland) Act 2003. However, there are some valuable benefits of membership of Paddle Scotland: *www.paddlescotland.org.uk*
- Go Paddling is a great resource for route-planning: *www.gopaddling.info*
- Know what to do in an emergency – #BeAdventureSmart: *www.adventuresmart.uk*
- If you are unsure about a new location, go with a local guide.
- If in doubt, don't go out!

ACKNOWLEDGEMENTS

Thank you to all the wonderful contributors who so kindly shared their stories with me. I am so grateful to you for your courage, honesty, time and wisdom. You will inspire and encourage so many people.

Thank you to Sara Jayne Kennedy for allowing me to use your valuable research.

Thank you to my commissioning editor Kirsty Reade for taking a leap of faith with me into the wonderful world of stand-up paddleboarding books three times now. I am hugely grateful to all the Vertebrate Publishing team for their brilliant skills and belief in my ideas. In particular, thank you to Helen Parry for her patience and hard work.

To my sister Jane for being my writing role model.

To my dad for sharing your love of the sea and a welcoming home to start this new chapter.

To my boys Henry and Johnny, thank you for being brave with your lives and teaching me to be brave with mine. You will always be my greatest adventure and joy. It's an honour to be your mum.

FURTHER READING AND LINKS

USEFUL ORGANISATIONS

Above Water: *www.abovewater.org*
Academy of Surfing Instructors (ASI): *www.academyofsurfing.com*
Adventure Smart: *www.adventuresmart.uk*
AquaPaddle: *www.aquapaddle.org*
British Stand Up Paddle Association (BSUPA): *www.bsupa.org.uk*
Go Paddling!: *www.gopaddling.info*
Paddle UK: *www.paddleuk.org.uk*
RNLI: *www.rnli.org*
Royal Life Saving Society UK: *www.rlss.org.uk*

BOOKS

Dr Catherine Kelly, *Blue Spaces: How and Why Water Can Make You Feel Better* (Welbeck Balance, 2021)
Belinda Kirk, *Adventure Revolution: The Life-Changing Power of Choosing Challenge* (Piatkus, 2021)
Kelly McGonigal, *The Joy of Movement: How Exercise Helps us Find Happiness, Hope, Connection, and Courage* (Penguin, 2021)
Jo Moseley, *Stand-Up Paddleboarding in Great Britain: Beautiful Places to Paddleboard in England, Scotland and Wales* (Vertebrate Publishing, 2022)

Jo Moseley, *Stand-Up Paddleboarding in the Lake District: Beautiful Places to Paddleboard in Cumbria* (Vertebrate Publishing, 2024)
Wallace J. Nichols, *Blue Mind: How Water Makes You Happier, More Connected and Better at What You Do* (Little, Brown, 2014)
Fiona Quinn, *Ignore the Fear: One Woman's Paddleboarding Adventure, 800 Miles from Land's End to John o' Groats with a Fear of the Sea* (Lemon Publishing, 2019)
Caroline Williams, *Move!: The New Science of Body Over Mind* (Profile Books, 2021)

MAGAZINES

SUPboarder online magazine: *www.supboardermag.com*
SUP Mag UK: *www.standuppaddlemag.co.uk*

#SHEPADDLES

Paddle UK's #ShePaddles ambassador movement is on a mission to continue to close the gap between men's and women's and girl's participation in the paddle sports community. Each year the ambassador programme works with a group of inspirational women across England, Scotland and Wales who share their love of paddle sports with their communities on the water and via social media.

In 2020, Clare Rutter was Paddle Cymru's (Canoe Wales') first and at that time only #ShePaddles ambassador, and describes the programme as 'nothing short of phenomenal'. She told me:

> 'It unites and empowers women to be who they want to be and how they want to be among peers without judgement, mutually respected and encouraged and firmly pushing aside any lurking, perceived negativity. It particularly also helps to develop and deliver leaders, managers and innovators because of this support. #ShePaddles gives a sense of warm, welcoming open arms, a literal hug or what we in Wales call a "cwtch".'

www.paddleuk.org.uk
@clare_rutter.ba.hons